The Business of Menopause

by Bev Thorogood

Typesetting and cover design by Anna Richards www.design-by-anna.co.uk

What's it like working with Bev and Floresco Training?

Bev did an excellent job, feedback from the staff was that she was very approachable and knowledgeable and made them feel comfortable and at ease. Bev very quickly understood our Boden approach and fitted in really well. She was extremely flexible with the delivery of the session and flexed to accommodate our shift pattern needs. The managers sessions were pitched just right, equipping them to talk about menopause without embarrassment and breaking some of the myths.

I was very impressed with the amount of information Bev was able to share with us – in a short time – yet in an engaging and friendly manner.

It was a great session.

J P Boden Limited London

Buckles' Solicitors were lucky enough recently to have two of Bev's Menopause in the Workplace Seminars, one for ladies going through the menopause and one for their Managers. I would say both sessions were extremely worthwhile and informative. This is a subject that is not openly spoken about generally let alone in the workplace despite the fact that a lot of ladies experience and often struggle with the symptoms for quite some time without actually knowing what's happening. Bev made the two sessions interesting, and everyone was able to ask questions and share experiences. I comfortably recommend Bev and Floresco Training to other companies who want to raise awareness and understanding of the menopause.

Buckles Solicitors Peterborough

I recently attended 'Menopause Awareness Training – Coping with the Menopause Workshop' at RAF Wittering, delivered by Bev Thorogood. The workshop was extremely well presented and covered a wide range of issues from explaining the   stages of the menopause to the potential symptoms and treatments available.

It was refreshing to be able to talk about the menopause and the impact it can have on individuals both personally and professionally. It was equally reassuring to learn that I'm 'normal'.

As a result of the workshop I now have a better understanding of how I can deal with my own symptoms naturally but also what medical help is available if required. In addition, I also feel empowered not only to speak to my doctor about how to obtain treatment, but also to my line manager, who attended the employer session, should I have any concerns about how it may impact my work without fear of being dismissed as irrationally emotional. For far too long the menopause has been a taboo subject, particularly in the workplace. Menopause Awareness Training is a huge step towards breaking that taboo.

Emma S

I attended a training on menopause that Bev gave a few months ago. At 47, I had started to experience a number of symptoms that I wasn't sure were all related to the perimenopause so I felt that I needed to start investigating for myself!

Bev's training was very enlightening, useful and great fun – not easy with what many consider to be a difficult subject! Not only was it jam packed with factual information but also gave some great ideas on how to mitigate some symptoms in a natural way, alongside the traditional treatments available from your medical care provider.

Bev encouraged a very interactive session and it was great to be able to interrupt and ask questions to get the most out of her impressive knowledge bank.

All in all, I came away with a much greater understanding of what was happening to me and the options available.

Would thoroughly recommend Bev for any training needs you may have

Elaine R

Our managers recently attended Bev's training on Awareness of Menopause in the Workplace and had their eyes opened to the impact of menopause on women and the ways in which they can suffer at work. It has changed the way New College Stamford approaches the issues surrounding menopause in the workplace and is now factored into our approach to flexibility and making reasonable adjustments.'

Stamford and Peterborough College

I attended Bev's webinar the other week and was extremely impressed with her approach, knowledge, and professionalism. So, I therefore decided to have a private session with Bev to discuss the menopause and the options of medicines that were available to me.

I had been extremely interested in hearing more about the plant-based alternatives that were available, rather than the standard HRT which is widely used. I wanted something that had less side effects and which worked more in line with the body's natural hormones.

Bev was knowledgeable and was able to advise me how best to approach my GP to ensure I got the correct HRT for me. I went armed with information, which enabled me to clearly get my GP to listen why I wanted this form of HRT and for him to prescribe what I felt was best for me.

The GP listened to the information that I provided and sort further expertise in the field, which has now happily led to me being prescribed the plant-based alternative.

Thank you, Bev, I would have never been any the wiser if I had not attended your webinar and I am so grateful that I did. I was that impressed that two of my friends have already attended a further masterclass.

Bev … you're a star and I will not hesitate to recommend you in the future!

Debbie W

I had the pleasure of working with Bev to look at various aspects of my life, with an initial focus on the debilitating effects of the menopause which I had basically put up with for well over 2 years. Bev was extremely knowledgeable in this area, she was objective, empathic and supportive. After just one session I was able to make decisions that basically have changed my life. Bev's approach is as an enabler who guided me through my thought process, this is done so effectively with passion and challenge that consequently, I was able to further develop my self-awareness and rationality. As a result I have been able to implement strategies and reasoning in both my home and work life.

Sessions are relaxed, warm and open, if this is your preferred coaching style, Bev is definitely the coach for you.

Lynda F

Foreword

Benjamin Franklin exclaimed that "in this world, nothing is certain except death and taxes" - testament to the fact that Ben was not the owner of a set of ovaries. If we are fortunate enough to live beyond our early 50's, then there is another certainty for us ovary owners – menopause.

Although menopause is a physiologically normal part of aging, for many people it can be a time of physical, psychological and emotional turmoil – a change from who we may have thought we were to a yet unknown version of ourselves. Navigating this transition requires good quality information to allow us to make the right choices for who we want to become.

In this book, Bev offers up to date, accurate information presented in an easily understandable style to help you steer your own unique path through the menopause. Information on managing symptoms, understanding what is happening in your body and how to manage your working life during this time are offered in a balanced and pragmatic way.

The menopause can offer us a unique opportunity to assess our lives and habits, change what no longer serves us and create a new way of being that will support us now and into older age. This book will help you reach the right decisions for you to move forward to the next phase of your life with grace and ease.

Dr Claire Macaulay MD, MBChB (Hons), MRCP, BSc(Hons)
Breast Cancer Oncologist and Somatic Sex Therapist
www.pleasurepossibility.com

Table of Contents

Warning

When I am an old woman I shall wear purple
With a red hat which doesn't go, and doesn't suit me.
And I shall spend my pension on brandy and summer gloves
And satin sandals, and say we've no money for butter.
I shall sit down on the pavement when I'm tired
And gobble up samples in shops and press alarm bells
And run my stick along the public railings
And make up for the sobriety of my youth.
I shall go out in my slippers in the rain
And pick flowers in other people's gardens
And learn to spit.
You can wear terrible shirts and grow more fat
And eat three pounds of sausages at a go
Or only bread and pickle for a week
And hoard pens and pencils and beermats and things in boxes.
But now we must have clothes that keep us dry
And pay our rent and not swear in the street
And set a good example for the children.
We must have friends to dinner and read the papers.
But maybe I ought to practise a little now?
So people who know me are not too shocked and surprised
When suddenly I am old, and start to wear purple.

Jenny Joseph

Preface

In Jenny Joseph's wonderful poem, Warning, she tells us of the outrageous things she will do when she is 'old', then beautifully forewarns that she may start sooner just to get her friends and family prepared for the shock.

In a world where so much emphasis is placed on youth, where the beauty industry presses women in their 20s to start using anti-wrinkle creams and female newscasters are cast aside at the sight of a first grey hair, Joseph's symbolic middle finger to society is refreshing.

I'm glad to say, I do believe that times are changing.

Middle aged women are coming into their own. They are no longer willing to sit back and be invisible.

Menopause isn't always fun but by heck it's better than the alternative and a privilage denied to many.

Alongside menopause, for most women, comes midlife.

That turbulent, indefinable and somewhat mystical time as we move through what I like to call all our 'midlife metamorphosis' – where we enter the chrysalis phase between the hungry caterpillar of our younger adult years, spent nibbling away at life, building a home, a family, a career – and into the glorious butterfly years where we emerge in vibrant, perfectly put together technicolour.

Unlike most primates, we women have the unique ability to continue to live long after our reproductive duties are finished. Dubbed the 'grandmother hypothesis' – this evolutionary development seems designed to help the elders 'alloparent' the young.

This is not surprising when we consider that alongside menopause comes knowledge, experience and wisdom. Unhindered by the baggage of our younger years, midlife is a time of exciting change and new beginnings – if we can just navigate our way through this bumpy middle ground.

Introduction

Midlife brings with it such a period of change. Physically we, as women, are undergoing myriad changes to our body; changes that affect not only how we look but also how we feel and how we perform in our job, how we manage our relationships and our social life. We may be dealing with changes in our environment, as children leave the nest or as we take on the role of carer for aging parents. We may be reaching a pinnacle in our career, taking on bigger projects, promotions and bringing all our knowledge and wisdom to our work.

However, we may also be dealing with changes in our ability to perform at work with the same ease and confidence, as peri-menopause kicks in and we begin to wonder if we're losing our minds. Our relationships can suffer as our energy drops, our confidence wanes, we no longer feel as sexy and physical changes can make intimacy uncomfortable.

And so, we say hello to menopause!

In past times it has been referred to as 'going through the change' – a term often disliked as being outdated and archaic. However, whether we like the terminology or not, we most certainly are going through major changes as we transition through menopause. Although I prefer to call it our midlife metamorphosis.

Reaching midlife seems to bring with it a need for some introspection. A time to reflect on the life we have lived so far and to look forward to the life yet to come. For some, we can find we have a greater disposable income and more time to ourselves in which to spend it. For others it can mean feeling trapped between caring for adult offspring unable to afford to leave home and elderly parents who, whilst living longer, may be struggling with conditions like dementia and Alzheimer's.

As women, we so often put the needs of others first. Let's face it, isn't that what society would have us believe being a good wife, mother, daughter, sister or friend is all about?

We may never have prioritised our own self-care, feeling guilty or selfish if we put ourselves first. We can feel lost and purposeless as the world around us moves on and we are left wondering how to fill the void. Uncertain of our new identity and confused about what the hell has happened to the person we used to be.

Add to that the general lack of education around peri-menopause and we really can feel like an alien has invaded our world!

It's a common analogy - I've heard many midlife women liken these feelings to the film Alien – like a parasite has invaded their being and is taking over their body and mind.

The image of menopause in the media doesn't help much either. We're constantly reminded of how miserable a period in our life this is. Images of rosy cheeked women with sweat beading the overwhelming fuzz of hair that has suddenly decided to adorn the top lip (and the chin, and the chest!).

Often menopause is portrayed as something we simply have to endure in silence and carry around with us, like a ball and chain. It's embarrassing and humiliating and ....perfectly natural!

Whilst it is a natural process and one that 100% of women will go through, assuming they live long enough, it is also important to recognise that all women will experience their menopause differently. Some will sail through with barely a flutter while others will feel like they want to take on and fight every man, woman and child that comes within 100 feet.

I'll be discussing the biology behind menopause in a little more detail later in the book, so I don't want to get bogged down in the hows and the wherefores right here, but suffice to say that whether you sail through or feel every menopausal bump in the road, making positive changes to your lifestyle habits will have immediate and long-lasting benefits to your health and quality of life.

I can say this with absolute conviction because I know first-hand how eating a diet rich in all the essential nutrients the body needs, ensuring the body gets to move about as a body is designed to, sleeping well and managing stress can significantly improve or even eliminate peri-menopausal symptoms.

Like many women hitting midlife, I began to see changes in my body – my weight was getting out of control, I was tired and quite frankly feeling old and frumpy. I had only one goal in mind. To shed the excess pounds that had somehow found their way to my waistline, so that I could wear the clothes I wanted to wear. That was it. I genuinely believed that losing weight was going to be the answer to all my feelings of inadequacy – from my ever-declining self-esteem to my complete loss of libido.

I was wrong.

Whilst shifting my unwanted weight certainly helped on the surface, the most profound benefits ran much deeper than simply the cosmetic changes.

I worked on much more than my diet. I started to

prioritise exercise and movement again and my strength, flexibility and achy joints started to improve.

I worked on my personal growth. I started to meditate. Began journaling. Practiced gratitude and I hired a personal coach to help me work out who I wanted to be for the rest of my life!

My mindset shifted. I started to view the world around me differently. I started to question some of the deeply held beliefs I'd carried with me my whole life and I started to look at getting older differently.

However, despite all of my best efforts at looking after my health, I still had some persistent symptoms that simply would not shift and on top of that, I was really struggling in my job.

I had always believed (mistakenly I now realise) that HRT was out of the question for me as my mum died from breast cancer when she was 54 (I was 22). It wasn't even something I had considered as I was convinced my risk was too high and I would never have been prescribed it. So, for quite some time I struggled on with ever worsening symptoms, including anxiety, high stress, poor memory, poor concentration and generally muddy thinking.

I've always prided myself on my memory – yes, I'd occasionally forget little things, but generally speaking I remember stuff. I used to laugh at my husband's need to write lists of lists. The way he would leave his car keys inside his lunch box so he wouldn't forget to take his packed lunch to work! But not me, I didn't need silly little reminders. My memory was rock solid.

At least it was, until peri-menopause kicked in.

I remember when I was about 51 I had the most

embarrassing moment while I was working for the Ministry of Defence.

Here's the story, or at least the bits I remember!

I had walked from my office to our purchasing department clutching a purchase order for some metal racking. It was a biggish order, amounting to around £4800. I'd chatted to the purchasing clerk and asked her to place the order for me.

When I returned to my office, I briefly mentioned to my boss that I'd just put the order in for the racking. His response caught me off guard. He told me he'd seen the racking and it looked great, and the "lads in the workshop were very happy with it".

I was totally confused. "How can they be happy with it? What do you mean you've seen it? I've only just this minute placed the order". He now looked as confused as me.

"It was delivered last Friday" he told me. "It's been assembled and it's full of kit now".

Today was Tuesday. How on Earth could the kit have been delivered four days before I'd even ordered it. It was a total mystery.

I checked back through my records to discover that I'd placed the order myself, online, at 7.30am the Monday of the week before. I had no recollection of placing the order, although all my paperwork was as it should have been. The only way I knew I'd actually placed the order was by checking back through my Google history and my emails.

To this day I have no recollection of placing the order, despite having very clear, physical evidence to show that I did.

I don't know if you've ever experienced anything similar but let me tell you it scared me. A lot!

I felt like I was losing my mind. I felt incompetent. I

felt stupid. In fact, I was mortified.

I was fairly new to this particular role and I was convinced my boss must have been wondering what kind of idiot he'd recruited.

Thankfully, that's the worst episode of brain fog and memory loss I've had, although I still find that I don't feel quite as 'sharp' as I used to be.

It was episodes like the story I shared above that finally convinced me to revisit HRT and to find out the real facts rather than the sensationalist newspaper headlines I'd been guided by previously.

I suppose what I'm trying to get across, is that depending upon the severity of your menopausal symptoms, you may not be able to eradicate them through lifestyle changes alone and HRT may well be the best course of treatment for you. The decision to medicate or not is yours and yours alone and there is no right or wrong decision.

In this book I will give you information on medical, non-medical and lifestyle changes that will help guide you through the options available to give you the best chance to have a positive menopause and a long, healthy, independent old age.

The population is living longer, with the average life expectancy of a woman in the UK being just over 82 years, so we need to be starting early to make sure that we can enjoy our old age free from as many preventable illnesses as possible.

My guidance and advice is based on a holistic approach to health. What I mean by that is that it's much more than just what we eat and how much we exercise. Good health incorporates mind, body and spirit and my NESST Model aims to bring all of these elements into balance.

Before I go any further, I want to manage your expectations a little here. I don't think it's necessary that you have to understand in detail all the biology of how the body works in order to effectively manage your menopause but having a basic understanding of what is happening as we head towards it helps to explain WHY it's good to make these lifestyle changes rather than simply being told WHAT you should be doing.

I also think by having a basic understanding of the science you can make far better, well informed choices around how you manage your menopause transition.

I've tried to make it as user friendly as possible so that you can easily digest the fundamentals. I feel it's important that you at least know the basics, especially if you need to speak to your GP.

I believe many women reaching midlife get to a crossroads at which point they stop and take stock of their life. This certainly happened for me. Which is why I want to encourage you to see this time in your life not as being in the 'midst of a miserable menopause' but as the start of a brand new, exciting chapter.

That's why my NESST model incorporates mindset as well as physical health.

Throughout the book I give you pointers and tools to help evaluate your current reality and put in place strategies to feel more positive about menopause and midlife in general.

Full of common sense, practical tips and tools, you will discover that I am unapologetically middle of the road in my approach to health and wellbeing. I don't do extremes – so unless you have a medical or religious reason to eliminate certain things from your life, nothing is banned. The body is a finely tuned, well balanced piece of equipment and I strongly believe that when you adopt an extreme approach in one area then there will inevitably be a corresponding payoff somewhere else. And it's normally not for the better.

I believe in moderation – I know, not very sexy right? But I also strongly believe that when we adopt a moderate, pragmatic approach to habit change, those changes become easier to sustain long term, with fewer relapses and a far higher success rate. It's also just a lot easier and less restrictive to know that you can have pretty much anything you want, so long as you have it in moderation.

The book is intended to be a practical, helpful guide to navigating your menopause transition and living a happier, healthier midlife. I would suggest you read it through fully at least once and then simply dip in and out of the various chapters as and when you need to remind yourself of those healthy behaviours.

As you go through the chapters, you'll be directed to additional resources that you can download as well as a useful contacts and resources section at the end of the book.

At any time, as you go through the pages of this book, you can reach out to me by email at bev@florescotraining.co.uk or come and join my fabulous Facebook community Your Best Midlife where you'll be surrounded by other amazing women making the very best of their midlife. Surrounding yourself with the right social network is a powerful way to make successful changes in your life.

I wanted to finish off this introduction with a bit of an explanation as to why I feel so strongly that women need to feel supported in the workplace.

After 2 years of struggling with symptoms including

anxiety, stress, low mood, tearfulness, brain fog, night sweats and hot flushes I knew I needed to make some changes. I did not, at that time, understand that the anxiety, stress and brain fog were symptoms of menopause.

Like many women in their late 40s and 50s I had a number of other, non-work-related, issues in my life that were adding to my overwhelm. My daughter had a very traumatic labour giving birth to my granddaughter and was constantly in and out of A&E for the next 2 years as the medical practitioners tried without success to identify the cause of her condition. Apart from the inevitable worry this was causing, I was also taking on child-care responsibilities as a consequence.

My husband, Mark, was leaving the Royal Air Force after 38 years and the life we'd known for the 25 years we'd been together was about to be completely turned upside down. Would he be able to get another job at the age of 55? How long would we be financially secure if he couldn't get work?

My father-in-law had terminal cancer and was a 3-hour drive away.

On top of all that my sister-in-law had moved into the house right next door to Mark and I as she had suffered brain damage from a diabetic coma following the amputation of her foot. Mark was her primary carer which placed an incredible strain on us all.

Whilst my circumstances are unique to me, the additional strain placed on midlife women (and men too of course) is not uncommon and often runs hand in hand with the onset of peri-menopause. It's difficult to clearly know whether the anxiety we may experience is a result of life stresses or linked to menopause or other events. Unfortunately, GPs are often quick to prescribe anti-depressants which have been shown to be less effective that HRT or talking therapies when it comes to menopausal depression and low mood.

Going back to my personal story, after 2 years of struggle I finally asked my boss if he would support an application for me to take 12 months unpaid leave from the Ministry of Defence.

I felt that 12 months would be enough time to get myself back on track. Mark would have sorted out his next career, my daughter (hopefully) would have had her medical issues resolved. Sadly we knew my father-in-law and possibly my sister-in-law were unlikely to live more than 12 months so I felt that after a period of leave I'd be in a better position to return to work.

Sadly, despite having always been a reasonably high performer with over 30 years' exemplary service, my request was rejected on the grounds of financial constraints.

I made the decision to resign from my job in March 2018 as I just couldn't see how I could continue.

Unfortunately, at that time there was no training to help either managers or colleagues recognise that what I was dealing with was peri-menopause. At no point was I referred to occupational health. Most probably because I wasn't aware that much of what I was dealing with was menopause-related, and I never asked for any help.

There was no formal menopause policy in place. I was not given an exit interview and therefore I was never able to explain properly what I was dealing with. My manager was exceptionally supportive, but he had not had any menopause awareness training either and at just 27 years old, I doubt he could really comprehend what I was going through.

It is somewhat ironic that just a few months after I left the Ministry of Defence and my role working for the Royal Air Force, a chance conversation with an ex-colleague led to me being invited to deliver some menopause awareness training for staff at the Royal Air Force's Head Office at Air Command in High Wycombe.

I am glad to say that the Civil Service in the UK now has a comprehensive menopause policy which is accessed by the Ministry of Defence, and I was later contracted to deliver menopause awareness training at a number of Royal Air Force Stations across the UK as part of an ongoing programme by RAF Air Command.

At the time of writing this book I have worked with dozens of organisations across all sectors and delivered menopause awareness training to thousands of employees. I am committed to raising awareness of the impact of menopause on working women and to support businesses to create an environment where women and men feel supported and confident that they can access the help they need to remain productive and happy in their work.

I wholeheartedly believe that the most effective way to help retain valuable female talent within the workplace is to ensure that menopause is spoken about openly and without fear of judgement.

Greater awareness of what menopause is, when and why it happens, and the impact of symptoms can help reduce stigma and ensure that those struggling are able to ask for, and access, the help they need so that they can remain a valuable asset to the organisation.

CHAPTER 1

66 So many women I've talked to see menopause as an ending. But I've discovered this is your moment to reinvent yourself after years of focusing on the needs of everyone else. It's your opportunity to get clear about what matters to you and then to pursue that with all of your energy, time and talent. 99

Oprah Winfrey — American TV Personality

1 What is Menopause

The word *menopause* comes from Greek origin and was originally termed by the French in the 1800s. It essentially means the pausing (or cessation) of the female menses (periods or 'monthlys').

Menopause is classed as just one day in a woman's life – the day 12 consecutive months from the date of her last period – so a woman will only know retrospectively that she has reached menopause. This is the date at which medically she's classed as no longer producing eggs and therefore no longer fertile.

Before that date, and during her normal reproductive years, she is classed as *pre-menopausal* and after that date, until the day she dies, she is *post-menopausal*.

Peri-menopause, which essentially means 'around the time of' menopause, starts when the female body begins its journey towards menopause. It is during this peri-menopausal phase that a woman's monthly cycle may change as the main hormones responsible for reproduction begin to decline and fluctuate.

This peri-menopausal time is when many of the symptoms associated with menopause start to rear their heads. It can occur up to 10 years prior to that one day of menopause and symptoms may last for a few years into post-menopause for some women.

Menopause usually occurs between the age of 45 to 55 for most women, with the average age in the UK being 51.

When a woman reaches menopause between 40 and 45 it is classed as an early menopause.

For women who go through menopause under the age of

40 the term most often used is *Premature Ovarian Insufficiency (POI)* and this condition occurs for approximately 1 in 100 women and can happen to women as young as their teens.

Premature menopause may also be triggered by either surgical or medical intervention, for example where a younger woman has had surgery to remove the womb and/or the ovaries as well as those who may be undergoing certain cancer treatments.

To summarise, *Menopause* is one day, *pre and post menopause* refer to the time before and after that one day and *peri-menopause* refers to the period leading up to menopause as the sex organs begin their journey towards no longer being able to reproduce. Early menopause can be spontaneous, known as *Premature Ovarian Insufficiency*, or it can be medically or surgically induced.

CHAPTER 2

" If you deal with it in a healthy fashion then I think you come out the other side a better person. I've got so much more energy now than I ever had in my early 50s before the menopause. "

Julie Walters – English Actress

2 A Quick Biology Lesson

It may be helpful to know where it all begins to help us understand where it ends!

As girls reach puberty, usually in their early teens, their body goes through a number of changes, including an increase in the amount of reproductive hormones; oestrogen and progesterone. These two hormones (among others) are responsible for maintaining the reproductive cycle, leading to menstruation each month. This cycle is usually somewhere between 28 to 32 days for most women.

During this period an egg is released around mid-month, known as *ovulation*.

The lead up to ovulation is known as the follicular stage during which rising levels of Follicle Stimulating Hormone (FSH) trigger the release of oestrogen to prepare the womb to receive an egg in preparation for pregnancy.

At the point of ovulation, usually around day 14 of the cycle, increases in levels of progesterone, along with a complex mix of other hormones, including luteinising hormone, cause the release of an egg from the ovaries.

The egg remains receptive to fertilisation by a sperm for about 24 hours.

If the egg is fertilised, progesterone remains high to support the egg through pregnancy. If the egg is not fertilised, oestrogen and progesterone start to fall which triggers the lining of the womb to be shed, resulting in what we recognise as a period. This later stage of the menstrual cycle is known as the luteal phase.

For most women, the menstrual cycle will continue from puberty until they reach menopause and is generally a fairly regular affair. Some women may find that they don't have regular periods and even for those women who do have regular monthly periods, their fertility can be impaired due to other reasons.

In general, women begin to see changes in their menstrual cycle as they begin to enter their peri-menopausal stage of life. Menstrual changes could be a change in frequency or a change in menstrual flow, with many women experiencing extreme bleeding.

Once a woman has been period-free for 12 consecutive months plus one day, she is classed as having gone through menopause and is referred to as post-menopausal.

The Role of Hormones

Hormones are chemical messengers that work in tandem with the nervous system to maintain the processes and systems within the body.

Whilst we tend to joke about women and their hormones, men have hormones too! However, due to the female body's ability to reproduce, and the fact that a woman's body changes throughout life as they come into and out of their reproductive years, the impact of these changes creates fluctuations in hormone levels that are generally more extreme than for men.

The body is always looking for what is known as *homeostasis*, which simply means it wants to be in balance. When our hormones fluctuate they can cause corresponding imbalances with other hormones resulting in changes in how the body works. These hormonal imbalances can manifest as physical, psychological or emotional symptoms.

The main hormones responsible for reproduction

are *oestrogen, progesterone and testosterone* although there are many other hormones that play a part in regulating the reproductive cycle.

When we understand the role of each of these key hormones the symptoms encountered by women as they go through puberty, menstruation and menopause make much more sense.

Oestrogen

Oestrogen, also spelled estrogen in American English, is the main player in terms of the female reproductive process but it also plays a far greater role in many different functions in the body.

We have oestrogen receptors on our cells all through our body, from our brains to our breasts. Oestrogen, as we've already mentioned, is responsible during the menstrual cycle for triggering ovulation, but it also has many other roles.

Oestrogen is involved in heart function, brain function, bone cell renewal, regulating cholesterol and lubricating body tissues.

There are 3 types of oestrogen produced in the body:

Oestrodial – the main form of oestrogen which is produced in the ovaries, is the predominant hormone involved in reproduction. When a woman enters peri-menopause it is this form of oestrogen than declines.

Oestrone – this form of oestrogen is produced in the ovaries but to a lesser degree than oestrodial. As oestrodial declines during peri-menopause, oestrone becomes the more dominant oestrogen, and once the ovaries stop functioning at menopause, production starts to take place in the fat cells, the liver and the adrenal glands.

Oestriol – is mainly produced in the liver in small amounts and is also produced by the placenta during pregnancy.

As oestrogen levels drop post-menopause, oestrone becomes the dominant oestrogen but in smaller amounts than that produced by the ovaries pre-menopause. The impact of low oestrogen levels on long term health is discussed in Chapter 3.

Progesterone

Progesterone is primarily responsible for supporting and nurturing the egg during fertilisation and into pregnancy.

Along with oestrogen, progesterone is produced in the ovaries as well as in the placenta during pregnancy.

Progesterone impacts on sleep, mood and pain tolerance and falling levels of progesterone in the luteal phase of menstruation and during peri-menopause can cause low mood and tearfulness.

Progesterone is involved in triggering the release of the lining of the womb, known as the endometrium, resulting in what we recognise as a period.

Synthetic forms of the hormone progesterone are called progestogen, or progestin in America, and are used in contraceptive medications and some hormone replacement therapy preparations.

Testosterone

Whilst we tend to think of testosterone as being a male hormone, women also produce testosterone. In fact, younger women produce more testosterone in the ovaries than they do oestrogen, however they convert most of the testosterone into oestrogen.

Much like it does for men, testosterone helps to support a woman's libido and enables her to enjoy a more satisfying sexual experience. It is also important for metabolic function, helping to support muscle growth, liver function, heart health and cognitive function. Testosterone helps with improved mood and increased confidence.

As well as the 3 sex hormones mentioned above, other hormones can be impacted as our hormone levels change.

Imagine our body as a seesaw. When our body is in balance the seesaw is perfectly still and parallel to the ground. But imagine the 3 sex hormones are sitting on the left hand seat of the seesaw and as they start to fall so the left hand side of the seesaw begins to drop towards the ground. The seat on the right-hand side begins to rise and everything becomes out of balance.

Whilst this is a hugely over-simplified analogy, it helps explain what happens in the body. Here are some other key hormones that can be knocked out of balance as oestrogen and progesterone levels fluctuate:

Cortisol – is a steroid hormone involved in the stress response. Released from the adrenal glands it is one of our 'fight or flight' hormones and is very good at keeping us safe and getting us out of trouble. However, when cortisol is chronically raised over an extended period of time it can have a negative impact on health, causing inflammation in the cells and reducing our immune response. The body is less able to metabolise fat as a fuel when cortisol is released which can also lead to weight gain and sugar cravings.

Melatonin – known as the sleep hormone, melatonin is responsible for letting the brain know that it is time to rest.

Triggered by darkness it helps prepare the body for sleep. A lack of melatonin can lead to insomnia and disturbed sleep. Artificial light, especially from backlit electronic devices, can interrupt the production of melatonin and lead to poor sleep.

Serotonin – is a complex hormone that impacts many areas of the brain including learning and development, memory and other cognitive functions such as reward and pleasure. However, it is generally recognised as a mood hormone, involved in levels of happiness and feelings of wellbeing.

Dopamine – is a neurotransmitter which means it transports information from the body to the brain. Dopamine is often referred to as the feel-good hormone as it triggers pleasure receptors in the brain linked to actions and rewards.

Thyroxine – is one of our metabolic hormones involved in maintaining energy levels (or metabolic rate), our heart and our digestion. Low levels of thyroxine can lead to low energy and weight gain.

Insulin – is used by the body to facilitate the conversion of sugar into energy. Released by the pancreas, insulin regulates the levels of blood sugar in the body. When blood sugar levels are high for an extended period of time complications such as poor circulation, eye problems and liver failure can occur. When blood sugar levels drop too low, a state known as hypoglycaemia, a person can rapidly become disorientated, confused and potentially fall into a diabetic coma which could lead to death.

There are many other hormones within the body. They are, effectively, our chemical messengers sending messages to the brain via the nervous system to maintain body functions.

They work on either a negative or positive feedback system, with more or less being produced depending upon the feedback received.

Anne-Marie's Story

At the age of 41 I began to have mood swings and ever-changing symptoms of heavy periods, dreadful night hot flushes and severe lack of sleep. Sometimes getting only two hours per night. I would wake up exhausted and this was causing a cumulative effect of a whole host of symptoms. I didn't realise that I was probably already a long way into my perimenopause journey. My monthly cycle went from 6 weeks to 4 weeks, to 2 weeks back to 5 weeks and then over the next two years I began missing monthly cycles altogether. I would suffer really heavy and very irregular cycles and spotting until my GP sent me for womb biopsies and ultrasound scans. These all came back clear and my symptoms just got worse. I was a Police Officer and qualified teacher at the time and was training new recruits, and I would stand in the classroom for some 5-6 hours a day. I felt ill and exhausted most days and this was further compounded by the fact that with every hot flush I felt like I was going to keel over as I was so light headed and heavy legged. I repeatedly attended my GP on numerous occasions whereby I was given medication that was actually ordinarily prescribed to regulate blood pressure to see if it would help with the hot flushes. I was also given three different lots of anti depressants, none of which did anything at all for my low mood or hot flushes. My GP openly admitted that they get very little training in menopause. I was finding every day a complete struggle and I didn't know how I could possibly carry on working and nearly quit on three occasions. However, after speaking with my Occupational Health

Department I was pleasantly surprised to find how supportive they were. They would offer to reduce my hours in the working day and allow me to work from home whenever I should be having a really bad patch. I aired my concerns to my GP regarding my mothers history of suffering from endometrial cancer and asked if it would be safe for me to receive HRT. They couldn't really give me a straight answer. I ended up undertaking training courses and wellness qualifications to try to understand more myself and it helped a little but I wanted to hear confirmation from a trained medical professional. It was at this time I contacted a menopause specialist GP and was given the information I needed. I was informed that I would be at no more risk of getting endometrial cancer than someone who drinks excess alcohol or who is overweight. I have been taking Estrogen, progesterone and testosterone for women and have to say it has completely changed my life, it's the best thing I have ever done and will continue to do so. I now listen to and help women on a personal level going through symptoms of menopause as I feel it's extremely important for them to get the true picture and to understand that they are not alone in their journey. I had lost my complete zest for life and was completely overwhelmed and I know plenty of women in the same boat. I'm thankful to say I now feel much better and I wish I'd have had personal support for coping with the crippling effects on day to day existence. Just having someone to talk to who understands can really help.

CHAPTER 3

66 I see menopause as the start of the next fabulous phase of life as a woman. Now is a time to "tune in" to our bodies and embrace this new chapter. If anything, I feel more myself and love my body more now, at 58 years old, than ever before. 99

Kim Catrall - Actress

3 When Does Menopause Happen

The average age for a woman to go through menopause in the UK is 51. The normal expected age range is between 45 and 55 although some women may be older than this.

As mentioned previously there is a condition known as Premature Ovarian Insufficiency (POI) which affects a smaller, although not insignificant, number of women under the age of 40. In fact, approximately 1% of women will go through a natural, spontaneous menopause under the age of 40. About 1 in 1000 women will experience POI under the age of 30 and around 1 in 10,000 under the age of 20.

The term POI is also sometimes called premature ovarian failure, although this is not entirely accurate as in some cases the ovaries do not fail completely but fluctuate in their ability to produce an egg or sufficient sex hormones.

For women who are diagnosed with POI there can be psychological pain as they come to terms with their potential infertility. Help and support can be found through a charity called The Daisy Network in the UK which offers advice and support as well as up to date research to women affected by POI. Their website can be found at www.daisynetwork.org.

Some women will experience a premature menopause as the result of surgical or medical intervention.

When a woman undergoes a hysterectomy (where the womb is removed) or an oopherectomy (where one or both ovaries are removed) she will stop having periods, but may also experience the onset of menopausal symptoms. This may or may not have been explained to her by her consultant, and may, in some cases, come as a complete surprise.

Certain cancer treatments, including chemotherapy and

radiotherapy treatments, can bring on menopausal symptoms due to either permanent or temporary damage to the ovaries, and again, this may be a shock to a patient who has not been informed this could happen.

Whilst we stereotypically think of menopausal women as being older, middle aged women close to retirement, as we can now see, menopause can affect women of all ages. It is really important that we don't pigeonhole women – never make an assumption that a woman is too young to be menopausal.

There is often a familial similarity in when a woman goes through menopause – if your mum had an early menopause there is an increased expectation that you, too, will experience an early menopause. However, this is not always the case. There really are few definitives when it comes to menopause.

A large-scale study carried out by the University of Queensland on 50,000 post-menopausal women concluded that girls who begin menstruating under the age of 12 are at a greater likelihood of going through an early menopause. However, once again, this is not always the case.

The study also found that women who didn't have children were more likely to go through menopause earlier than those who do.   But this also is not always the case.

The key message here is, I believe, that there may be factors that could affect how soon a woman reaches menopause, but there are very many 'exceptions to the rules' and therefore it is difficult to state categorically that one factor will affect another.

CHAPTER 4

" All of a sudden I don't mind saying to people, 'You know what? Get out of my life. You're not right for me.' It's wonderful and liberating. "

Whoopie Goldberg - Actress

4 The Symptoms

When we think of a menopausal woman we tend to imagine a middle aged woman wafting herself frantically with any piece of cardboard she can get hold of!

What we are imagining is the archetypal 'hot flush' (also known as a hot flash). But hot flushes are just one of many symptoms related to menopause. In fact, there are 34 recognised symptoms that can be directly attributed to the changing hormones during peri-menopause and into post-menopause, although there could be many more 'symptoms of symptoms'.

These 34 symptoms can be broken down into 3 main areas:

Physical

Psychological

Emotional

Whilst the symptoms may seem totally random, ranging from migraines and brain fog to urinary infections and dry eyes, when we consider the role of the hormones, particularly oestrogen, in the wider functions of the body, they make a bit more sense.

Let's look at what these 34 symptoms are.

Physical:

Hot flushes (flashes) and Night Sweats (vasomotor system issues)

Irregular periods (changes in frequency, duration and flow including excessive bleeding or 'flooding')

Vaginal dryness and thinning of the tissues around the vaginal and urethral areas causing pain, especially during intercourse

Migraines and headaches

Joint aches and pains

Itchiness and dry skin – some women complain of a feeling of insects crawling under their skin, a condition known as 'formication'.

Thinning hair and brittle nails

Breast tenderness

Burning mouth

Digestive discomfort including indigestion, bloating, constipation, diarrhoea and stomach cramps

Gum problems and a metallic taste in the mouth

Weight gain – often related to changing hormones, but also due to a natural slowing of the metabolism as we get older

Insomnia and sleep disturbances

Urinary Tract Infections (UTIs)

Urge and stress incontinence

Heart palpitations

Allergies

Body odour changes

Dry eyes

Psychological:

Anxiety

Depression

Panic attacks

Poor concentration

Memory disturbances

Cloudy thinking (sometimes called 'brain fog')

Loss of confidence and self-esteem

Loss of libido

Emotional:

Irritability

Low mood

Tearfulness

Short temper

In the longer term a lack of oestrogen post-menopause can affect bone density, potentially leading to osteoporosis as well as an increased risk of heart disease and dementia.

So, as you can see, when we consider the role of oestrogen throughout the body, the wide range of symptoms begin to make more sense.

Oestrogen is involved in brain function and a lack of oestrogen can affect other hormones such as a serotonin, dopamine and melatonin, all of which can create cognitive issues such as brain fog, anxiety, depression, insomnia and poor memory. These changes are what cause some of the emotional symptoms such as low mood, tearfulness and irritability.

Oestrogen helps to maintain body tissue and acts as a natural cell lubricant therefore a lack of oestrogen can cause itchiness and soreness, especially in the more delicate areas such as the vagina, urethra, skin and eyes.

The digestive system is extremely susceptible to hormone changes and fluctuations in oestrogen levels can cause bloating and digestive irritation.

Oestrogen receptors are located all over the body so it makes sense that as oestrogen levels change the impact may be felt in a diverse range of symptoms.

Do All Women Get Symptoms?

Thankfully not all women will experience symptoms. Approximately 1 in every 4 women will sail through their menopause with barely any noticeable symptoms at all, they'll simply realise they've not had a period for more than 12 months and may wonder what all the fuss is about!

However, the majority of women will experience some symptoms in varying degrees of frequency, severity and type.

About 25% of women will experience severe and often life changing symptoms and for these women it can be a miserable time in their life. They may very well require additional support within the workplace and are the most likely to leave their job as a result of their menopausal symptoms.

For the 50% of women in the middle of the two extremes above, symptoms may come and go and change over time. They may need occasional support to help with a short-term symptom or they may find they can manage their symptoms well enough without needing to ask for additional help.

It is imperative that we recognise that no two women will experience their menopause in the same way and we cannot, therefore, offer a one size fits all solution when it comes to workplace support.

When Do Symptoms Start

Symptoms can begin as soon as peri-menopause starts as this is the point at which oestrogen and progesterone levels begin to decline.

For many women the first visible symptoms may be subtle changes in their menstrual cycle. They may also begin to encounter some of the psychological and emotional symptoms, such as mood swings and increased anxiety.

Often these symptoms creep up quite insidiously and many women find it difficult to put their finger on exactly what is changing. They may just say they 'don't feel like themselves' or they're 'losing the plot'.

Often, because peri-menopause can begin up to 10 years prior to menopause, women aren't expecting the cause of how they're feeling to be due to menopause. Peri-menopause could, in theory, begin as young as mid to late 30s and yet menopause would still fall within the normal age bracket of 45-55 years. At this point menopause is not usually on a woman's radar, or that of their GP for that matter.

Once again, we can see that all women experience menopausal symptoms in a unique way, and it is important that managers do not make assumptions about someone based on their age.

On the one hand we cannot assume that a woman is too young to be menopausal, as we now know that menopause can affect women of all ages.

On the other hand, we cannot assume that because a woman is of 'menopausal age' she will be symptomatic since we now know that a quarter of all women won't have symptoms.

The Longer-Term Health Implications of Low Oestrogen

Osteoporosis

Osteoporosis is a condition that results in a loss of bone density leading to brittle, fragile bones that break more easily. There are a number of risk factors associated with osteoporosis, including genetic predisposition, being of a low weight, some existing medical conditions, certain medications and in women, low levels of oestrogen.

Smoking and drinking alcohol can increase the risk factors associated with osteoporosis, which is also more prevalent in post-menopausal women than it is in men. Women of Caucasian or Asian origin have a higher risk of osteoporosis than women of Afro-Carribean origin due to bone size and density.

Some of the ways to reduce the risk of developing osteoporosis are discussed in later chapters when we look in more detail at exercise, nutrition and supplements.

Heart Disease

Women are 3 times more likely to die of heart disease than they are of breast cancer and whilst we often tend to think of heart disease as a man's issue, many women do suffer and their risk increases post menopause. Oestrogen is heart protective and up until menopause women generally have a lower risk profile for heart attack. However, post menopause, when the protective elements of oestrogen are dramatically reduced, our risk factors become similar to those of men.

Women often don't display the classic symptoms of a heart attack, there may be no chest pain or arm pain. Instead, they may feel a pain or tightness in the upper back and across the shoulders, they may feel nauseous, light-headed or dizzy, they may vomit or feel they have flu-like symptoms or put their discomfort down to acid reflux.

Stopping smoking, eating a healthy diet, exercising regularly, managing stress, maintaining a healthy weight and getting enough sleep can all help to reduce the risk of heart disease. Hormone Replacement Therapy has also been shown to reduce the risk of heart disease in post-menopausal women.

In addition, factors that can increase the risk of heart disease are things like high blood pressure, high cholesterol, obesity, diabetes and a family history of coronary heart disease.

We discuss lifestyle factors in greater detail later in the book.

Alzheimer's

According to Alzheimer's UK, 65% of those diagnosed with dementia are women, with Alzheimer's being the most common form of dementia.

Alzheimer's is caused by the build-up of amyloid and tau proteins in the brain and there appears to be a connection between falling oestrogen levels in post-menopausal women and an increased risk of developing Alzheimer's.

Research is still not clear on how or why this connection exists and there may be connections with other neurotransmitters such as serotonin, dopamine and acetylcholine. Studies have shown contradictory results with regard to the use of hormone replacements in preventing Alzheimer's. Alzheimer's UK cite concerns around the potential risks of HRT, including blood clots, breast cancer and stroke. However ongoing research around the use of modern, body identical HRT brings into question the validity of those concerns, which continue to reflect outdated data from an early study called the Women's Health Initiative in the early 2000s. I'll share more about that study later when I discuss hormone replacement therapy and risks.

CHAPTER 5

 One day you will look back and see that all along you were blooming.

Morgan Harper Nichols

5 Managing Menopause

Thankfully there are a number of ways in which women can help to alleviate some, if not all, of the symptoms associated with menopause. These can be broken down into 3 categories:

Medical

Non-medical

Lifestyle

We are going to look at each of these categories in more detail, but I should probably explain that these menopause management options do not necessarily stand alone and a combination of all 3 may well be the best solution for women in both the short and the longer term.

Certainly, there is little benefit in seeking out a medical solution if lifestyle factors are not addressed too. A blended approach is by far the best solution.

The Medical Route

I'm going to start with the medical route, because in my opinion when a woman's symptoms are severe the non-medical and lifestyle interventions may not offer an immediate enough solution to deal with the severity of the symptoms.

Hormone Replacement Therapy

Hormone Replacement Therapy has had something of a roller coaster ride in popularity since it was first introduced to women in the UK in 1965.

There was widespread evidence in medical literature that oestrogen successfully controlled menopausal symptoms but was also a key player in improving bone health and reducing the risk of osteoporosis, reducing the risk of heart disease, colon cancer and latterly dementia.

In 1993, a large clinical trial known as the Women's Health Initiative began which explored the health effects on women taking oestrogen only or combined HRT (oestrogen + progesterone).   This trial was prematurely stopped in 2002 following findings that women taking combined HRT showed an increased risk of breast cancer, heart disease, stroke and blood clots.

When the published findings from the prematurely terminated trial hit the media, the use of HRT for the management of menopausal symptoms dropped dramatically, among fears that women were at a high risk of breast cancer.

Between 2004-2007 the Women's Health Initiative results were re-investigated and it was assessed that many of the risks had been over-estimated, that the study subjects were, on average, in their mid-60s and often had a number of comorbidities.   They also found that in fact there were many additional benefits such as those already mentioned above.

The Risks Associated with HRT

The current guidance on HRT is that it is an effective, low risk treatment for most women starting medication under the age of 60.   The guidelines issued by the National Institute for Health and Care Excellence (NICE) state that the benefits of taking HRT outweigh the risks for the MAJORITY of women.

To put the risk in context, for every 1000 women in the UK aged between 50-55, around 23 of them will be diagnosed with breast cancer over the next 5 years. In women using combined HRT, an additional 4 women will be diagnosed with breast cancer. The risk of breast cancer in the group of women using HRT rises from 2.4% to 2.7%.

However, putting this into context, this risk is significantly lower than for women who smoke 10 cigarettes per day, drink alcohol or who are obese.

For women taking oestrogen only HRT there is no increased risk of breast cancer.

For women starting HRT over the age of 60 there is a very small increased risk of heart disease.

For women taking HRT in tablet form there is a very small increased risk of blood clot. There is no associated risk for women using transdermal (through the skin) HRT.

HRT is the most effective treatment for hot flushes, but it also has recognised long-term health benefits as follows;

- improved bone density means lower risk of bone fracture
- improved brain function means lower risk of dementia
- improved heart function means a lower risk of coronary heart disease
- lowers cholesterol
- reduced risk of Type 2 diabetes

Not to mention a lower chance of vaginal dryness and painful intercourse.

Types of HRT

There is a wide range of HRT available and it comes in various forms, dosages and 'routes of delivery' i.e. how it is administered:

- Orally in tablet form
- Transdermally (via the skin) through patches, creams, gels and, most recently, sprays.
- Implants under the skin

Progesterone can also be administered through the Mirena coil, an intrauterine device (IUD) implanted inside the womb that provides a slow release of hormones that act locally to protect the lining of the womb.

There are also vaginal oestrogen medications which are applied locally to the vaginal area either as a gel, a pessary or via a soft ring which is inserted into the vagina. Vaginal oestrogen carries no risk of clot or breast cancer and can be taken by women who are unable to take other forms of HRT.

The most common form of HRT is a tablet however, there is some evidence that transdermal application may have fewer negative side effects since it does not go through the digestive system and therefore does not impact the liver, where clotting agents are produced.

With such a wide array of HRT options available it is likely that it may take some months and a bit of trial and error to find the combination and application option most preferred by each individual. Often side effects will settle down after two to three months, therefore switching before then may not be beneficial.

For women who have a womb, combined HRT should be prescribed, since the addition of progesterone protects the lining of the womb, called the endometrium, from the possibility of endometrial cancer.

For women without a womb there is no need to prescribe progesterone and oestrogen only treatment can be prescribed. For oestrogen only HRT there is no increased risk of breast cancer.

Bio-Identical HRT or Body-Identical HRT?

Regulated, body identical HRT is available on prescription through the NHS in the UK. The majority of oestrogen prescribed is body identical which means it is derived from plant oestrogen and has a molecular structure identical to that found in the human body. At present, most progesterone is synthetic however there is one body identical progesterone licenced for use on the NHS and it is called Utrogestan. It is thought that micronized body identical progesterone has a lower risk for breast cancer than synthetic progestogens.

These regulated medications have undergone rigorous testing and their risks and ingredients will be fully documented.

Bio identical HRT on the other hand, is unregulated and is neither available via NHS prescription or recommended by NICE or The British Menopause Society.

Often bio-identical progesterone is prescribed as a progesterone cream. However, there is a question mark over whether this form of application allows for a sufficient amount of progesterone to be absorbed into the body to provide adequate protection to the lining of the womb.

Bio identical HRT is prescribed by private practitioners who will have the preparation prepared for you in what are known as compounding pharmacies. Bio identical HRT is expensive and may contain ingredients you are not aware of and the dose you actually receive may not be certain.

Whilst many women feel bio identical is a more 'natural' option and carries fewer risks, neither of these are true. Most regulated body identical HRT, as mentioned earlier, is plant based and comes from 'natural' sources. Unregulated bio identical HRT does not have to state the risks in the same way body identical regulated HRT has to, therefore whilst the risks may not be detailed, it does not mean the risks are not there.

The Myths Surrounding HRT

There are a number of myths and misunderstandings surrounding the use of HRT. Let's address them here.

Myth Number 1:
If you take HRT you're simply delaying the menopause
HRT does not put your menopause on hold. It simply manages the symptoms. If you stop taking HRT and you begin to experience menopausal symptoms, for example hot flushes, it is simply that you are now experiencing symptoms you would have been having anyway but they're no longer being managed. Some women continue to experience symptoms for many years after menopause. Coming off HRT can reveal symptoms that were previously managed.

Myth Number 2:
Natural remedies are better than HRT as they don't contain chemicals
Whilst many products may be marked up as 'natural' they may be unsafe for a number of reasons. Firstly most 'natural' products are unregulated and therefore their ingredients may be uncontrolled. Just because a product is derived from a plant does not mean it is risk free, there are many plant chemicals that are harmful to the body. Natural medicines may be contraindicated with other medications. If you do choose to opt for a 'natural' approach, it is wise to speak to a qualified medical herbalist who can prescribe safely.

Many HRT medications prescribed through your GP

are 'body identical' which means their structure is the same as the hormones in our body, and they are naturally derived from plant oestrogens (usually soy or yam) – all very 'natural'!

Myth Number 3:
You have to come off HRT after 5 years

If a woman is otherwise healthy, there is no medical reason why a woman needs to stop taking HRT after 5 years, and indeed there is evidence to suggest that there are long-term health benefits in taking HRT indefinitely. Think of it this way, if a person has Type 1 diabetes they supplement with insulin, because their pancreas fails to produce sufficient insulin. Therefore, if a women is peri or post-menopausal her ovaries fail to produce sufficient oestrogen, therefore supplementing with oestrogen meets that need. There are many women happily enjoying the benefits of HRT well into their 80s. That said, at present there is insufficient research to show the potential long-term risks associated with taking combined HRT indefinitely. It really comes down to doing your due diligence and making an informed decision based on your own assessment of the risks and benefits.

Myth Number 4:
Your symptoms need to be debilitating before you can be prescribed HRT

How severe a woman's symptoms need to be before she chooses to take HRT is absolutely down to personal choice. A woman has the right to decide when she feels the time is right to get help and she doesn't have to wait until her symptoms are severe. Women starting combined HRT under the age of 50 reduce their risk of developing breast cancer and there is growing evidence to show that starting HRT early can help provide protection from conditions such as osteoporosis, heart disease and dementia, so why would she wait?

Myth Number 5:
I can't take HRT while I'm still having periods.
Many of the symptoms associated with menopause start during peri-menopause, the period leading up to periods ending. It is during this peri-menopausal period that many women find they need relief from symptoms. There is also evidence to suggest that the younger a woman is when she starts taking HRT the lower the potential risks.

Antidepressants

Very often women experiencing anxiety, mild depression or low mood are offered anti-depressants by their GP. There is evidence to suggest that reproductive depression, as opposed to clinical depression, does not respond well to conventional anti-depressants such as Selective Serotonin Reuptake Inhibitors (SSRIs), for example Prozac.

Of course, there may well be women going through peri-menopause who also have clinical depression and antidepressants may be the right treatment. It is important to speak to a doctor who understands both menopause and depression well enough to be able to make the distinction. The NICE Guidelines state that HRT should be the first choice in treating menopausal depression, low mood and anxiety.

Women who cannot take HRT, either for medical or personal reasons, may be offered antidepressants to help with hot flushes and other vasomotor related symptoms.

There are also non-hormonal medications which may offer symptom relief, including Tibolone and Clonidine.

Psychological Therapies

Whilst not a medical intervention, there is strong research to show that talking therapies such as Cognitive Behavioural Therapy can have a positive effect on symptoms such as anxiety, stress and low mood as well as helping with some of the physical symptoms such as hot flushes and insomnia. CBT is a non-invasive therapy that helps the individual to manage their symptoms through their thought processes, offering exercises and tools to help manage thoughts, feelings and behaviour.

Further Help

There are some extremely good GPs out there, but sadly, there are also some that are not so up to date on their menopause knowledge. Often women feel uncomfortable challenging their GP, but doing a bit of personal research before booking an appointment can help.

Seeking out help from a menopause specialist can help to clarify the best treatment route for the individual.

The British Menopause Society website has a menopause specialist tool to help locate a specialist in your area and lists both NHS and private clinics.

There are also online specialists that can help including Dr Morton's – The Medical Helpline where, for a small monthly subscription, you can get easy access to a doctor or gynaecologist and you can also order your prescriptions directly from the site.

My Menopause Doctor is an online menopause advice

service provided by Dr Louise Newson. Dr Newson also offers private consultations at the Newson Health Menopause and Wellbeing Centre.

Or you can book a 60 minute consultation directly with me where we will discuss all aspects of your menopause management holistically, this will enable you to make an informed decision about the way you prefer to manage your menopause symptoms. You will have all the information you need to make decisions that work best for you, and the tools needed to get the best help, whether that's medical, non-medical or lifestyle related.

Preparing for a Visit to the GP

If you decide that a trip to the doctors is the right course of action for you, there are guidelines produced by the National Institute for Health and Care Excellence (NICE) in England (the devolved administrations in the UK may have their own guidelines), specifically relating to menopause, which GPs should be using to guide them towards the best course of treatment for their patients. Unfortunately, many GPs are unaware of these guidelines and are still advising and prescribing based on out-of-date information, often resulting from skewed data published following the Women's Health Initiative study.

The NICE Guidelines can be accessed through the NICE website or via the British Menopause Society website and there is a patient version which is a little easier to understand than the clinical guide. It is a good idea to download the guidelines, read through them and even take them with you to your GP appointment. The guidelines can also help you to prepare in advance so you are more likely to get the outcome you want from your appointment.

You can download a copy of my Menopause Action Plan from the resources section at the back of this book, which you can complete prior to visiting your GP.

The Non-Medical Route

Many women either cannot, or choose not to, go down the medical route to help with menopause symptoms and for those women there are alternative therapy treatments that they may wish to explore.

Whilst many of these therapies have little scientific evidence to support their efficacy, anecdotally many women find them helpful in treating menopausal symptoms; although none of them will replace lost oestrogen so may not provide the longer-term health protection that HRT will.

Herbal Medication

There are a number of herbs that may help with symptoms including things like red clover, black cohosh, sage, St John's Wort and evening primrose oil. Many of these supplements are available over the counter and from the internet although it is important to consider that supplements bought over the internet may not be produced from reputable sources and herbal medication is not currently regulated in the UK.

It is therefore advised that if a woman is looking to use herbal medication to treat her symptoms she seek advice from a registered medical herbalist. Details of registered medical herbalists can be found at the National Institute of Medical Herbalists website www.nimh.org.uk.

It should also be noted that many supplements are marketed as 'natural' alternatives to HRT. However just because something is called 'natural' does not necessarily mean it carries no risk – arsenic is natural!

Many herbal preparations are contraindicated with other medications and medical conditions. This is another good reason to seek help from a medical herbalist or to speak to your GP or pharmacist to check any herbal preparation doesn't conflict with other medication.

Complementary Therapies

Many women find that they benefit from some of the complementary therapies available. Again, there is little scientific research to suggest they work, however many women do find they help and it's worth trying different things to find out what does and doesn't work for each individual.

Here is a list of some complementary therapies that may help:

- Reflexology
- Aromatherapy
- Acupuncture
- Magnetic Therapy
- Hypnotherapy
- Reiki

The Research Council for Complementary Medicine has details of professional bodies relating to holistic and complementary therapy practitioners.
Visit www.rccm.org.uk

The Lifestyle Route

The information below relating to lifestyle habits to help with menopausal symptoms is, in reality, good advice regardless of age or gender. In fact, it's simply good advice for everyone. However, many of the poor lifestyle habits we can 'get away with' when we're in our 20 and 30s become more problematic as we head into our 40s and beyond.

Whilst HRT and/or any of the complementary therapies mentioned earlier can help, I can't stress enough the importance of including them as part of a healthy, well balanced lifestyle. It is not enough to simply treat the symptom without also addressing any negative habits that could have an impact on long term health and wellbeing.

In order to help understand what healthy lifestyle habits look like, I developed a very simple framework called NESST that includes all areas of health, including physical, psychological and emotional health.

Jenny's Story

I was diagnosed as being in menopause at the relatively early age of forty-two. I had only stopped taking the pill less than two years earlier and had been experiencing irregular and sometimes very painful periods. My sister suggested endometriosis (correct) and my mother suggested menopause (she was diagnosed at 43). Also correct. I burst into tears, much to the discomfiture of my rather awkward doctor. I don't think he had any idea why. I didn't want any more children, but I think the idea that a certain part of my life was over, was quite overwhelming.

He suggested HRT and, after some thought, I agreed. I had no contra-indications and nothing in my family medical history which would raise any red flags. I had been taking the contraceptive pill on and off (I had two children) since I was nineteen with no problems except regular, lighter, less painful periods. But I have low bone density (probably genetic) and the likely impact of an early menopause on my bones was a concern. So I took HRT for years until I was well into my fifties. I did consider taking it permanently, but I couldn't justify the cost. The endometriosis stopped, as did the occasional 'warm' feeling; these were my only menopause symptoms. By the way, I still get the 'warm' feelings and I'm now 68!

I know how lucky I am to have had such a straightforward menopause, and I know that it's not like this for everyone. But it does happen, and I hope it happens for you.'

CHAPTER 6

> The doctor of the future will give no medicine,
> but will instruct his patients in care of the human
> frame, in diet, and in the cause and prevention
> of disease.
>
> *Thomas Edison*

6 The NESST Framework

NESST is an acronym for the 5 pillars of health that includes Nutrition, Exercise, Sleep, Stress and Thoughts/Feelings (also often referred to as our mindset). It is a holistic approach to finding balance across mind and body – remember we talked about how the body likes to find homeostasis?

Nutrition

When it comes to eating well there is an absolute minefield of information which can lead to confusion and overwhelm. Faddy diets and fancy pills and potions can seem like the best solution but in reality, they're rarely sustainable and unlikely to be enjoyable.

The best diet is really about getting back to basics. Eating real food, in realistic portion sizes and aiming for a good mix of colours and textures.

We generally eat too much processed foods in our Western diets, sometimes because of convenience, sometimes because of a lack of knowledge or cooking skills. Changes in hormonal balance can lead to women craving carbohydrates and fast acting energy derived from sweet, sugary foods which can, of course, lead to unwanted weight gain as well as guilt and shame.

Here are some guidelines for a healthy diet:

- Aim to get 80% of food from whole, natural sources such as lean meat and fish, lots of different coloured fruits and vegetables (especially leafy greens), raw nuts and seeds, beans and pulses. Basically all the foods that come without a TV advert!
- Aim to limit processed foods and sugary snacks to less

than 20% of daily intake.

- Eat vegetables with every meal.
- Limit alcohol and caffeine consumption (especially if hot flushes and insomnia are an issue).
- Drink plenty of water, at least 2 litres per day (more if it's hot or you're very active).
- Eat protein and fats at breakfast and avoid sugary cereals.
- Eat slowly and purposefully, this will help with digestive issues and also reduce the chances of over-eating.

Women often gain weight during menopause due to changes in body composition and a slowing down of their metabolism. Learning to listen to hunger and fullness cues can help with weight management.

There is some evidence that eating foods rich in chemicals called phytoestrogens can help to support fluctuating hormone levels. Foods rich in phytoestrogens include soy products such as tofu, tempeh and edamame, oats, walnuts, flax (linseeds), apples, carrots, sesame seeds, lentils, barley and dried beans.

Managing Weight Gain

If weight gain is a worry, it is not a good idea to go down the very low calories, meal replacement diet route.

As we get older our metabolism slows down, this is true for men and women alike. Very low calorie diets cause a further slowing of the metabolism (correctly termed our metabolic rate) as the body has to adjust to taking in fewer calories. This is a double whammy for the metabolism and can result in low energy as well as side effects such as hair loss (also a symptom of menopause) and digestive issues (another menopause symptom). Therefore, very low calorie diets are simply going to exacerbate potential symptoms and are unsustainable in the long term.

Another factor to consider with highly restricted calorie plans, is that when you either reach your desired weight or get totally fed up of the restriction and return to a more realistic amount of calories, as you undoubtedly will need to, your metabolic rate (the speed at which you're able to use energy) is likely to have slowed down significantly. So much so that even if you are now eating fewer calories than you did before you started the diet, this will result in weight gain and you're likely to put on more weight than you started with.

The best way to lose weight safely and effectively is by reducing your calorie intake gradually to around 15–20% under your Total Daily Energy Expenditure (TDEE).

The TDEE consists of your basal metabolic rate – this is the number of calories required to maintain all bodily functions BEFORE we do any further activity, your non-exercise activity (ie general moving about during the day) plus any formal exercise.

This ensures that you are eating in a calorie deficit but not forcing your metabolism to slow too dramatically.

Let's quickly look at how to calculate your BMR + Activity to ascertain an estimate of your daily calorie needs.

To calculate your basal metabolic rate here is a simple equation for you to follow:

(10 × weight: kg) + (6.25 × height: cm) - (5 × age)-161

So for example, a 47 year old woman, weighing 81.6kg and 175cm tall would equate to:

(10×81.6) + (6.25×175) - (5×47) - 161 = 1983 kcal

This gives your basal metabolic rate, before adding in any exercise or activities. To calculate how active you are and to work out how many additional calories you are using through activity, we need to use an 'activity multiplier' as follows:

- Sedentary: little or no exercise = BMR x1.2
- Lightly Active: light exercise/sports 1-3 days/week = BMR x1.375
- Moderately Active: moderate exercise/sports 3-5 days/week = BMR x1.55
- Active: hard exercise/sports 6-7 days a week= BMR x1.725
- Extra Active: very hard exercise/sports and physical job = BMR x1.9

So for our example 47-year old woman with a BMR of 1983 who is pretty sedentary, maybe she has a desk job and doesn't take any additional exercise, her daily calorie needs would be *1983 x 1.2 = 2378 calories per day*.

If she then wanted to lose weight she would take 20% off that total giving her an estimated daily calorie intake of 1902 calories. You could take anywhere between 15-25% off by simply adjusting the equation. I wouldn't recommend taking more than 25%.

Many very low calorie diets limit calorie intake to just 600 or 800 calories per day which is simply not sustainable long term.

Of course, it will take longer to lose weight, but it is more sustainable, more pleasant and a much more healthy way to manage weight.

In order to speed up weight loss, our example woman could choose to maintain her calculated calories but add in more exercise, thus creating a greater calorie deficit whilst maintaining her metabolic rate.

Many women are concerned that hormone replacement therapy will lead to weight gain. There is no evidence to suggest that taking HRT will cause you to put on extra weight. In fact, what often happens is women begin sleeping better, they find they have more energy, feel more inclined to eat better and exercise and their weight is easier to manage.

In addition to managing energy intake through calorie tracking, there are other things that you can do to help with weight management. Here are a few tips that will help:

Eat Mindfully – often we try to multitask while we eat. The problem here is that we can end up consuming far more calories than we intend to (think how easy it is to keep dipping your hand into a big family bag of crisps when you're watching a movie!). Being mindful while eating can help us to be more aware of the amount of food we're consuming. Switch off the TV, put your mobile out of sight, put the book down and focus completely on the taste, the smell, the texture, the temperature, the colours and the setting of your food.

Slow Down – this is linked to being more mindful above. It takes some time for the hormones in the stomach to register that food is being consumed. By slowing down it gives the body a chance to catch up and gives the hormone leptin (the one that lets you know you're full and should stop eating) a chance to take effect. Slowing down can therefore help you to consume fewer calories and also aids the digestive process, reducing digestive issues and bloating.

Eat Smaller Portions - this may seem obvious but we're so much more conditioned to eat bigger portions than ever before. It's estimated that the average dinner plate is 30% bigger than it was 60 years ago. Restaurants offer all you can eat buffets and super-sized portions. We are surrounded by messages suggesting we should eat more. By simply choosing to use a smaller plate we can often reduce our calorie intake by up to a third. Go for smaller options in restaurants. By slowing down and being more mindful you'll find that a smaller portion will still satisfy your appetite.

Increase Exercise – the more you move around the more calories you will burn. The more muscle you have the more calories you will burn even at rest. I'll talk more about exercise in the next section.

Get enough sleep – sleep is one of the best kept weight loss secrets. When we are tired we are more likely to crave calorie dense, sugary, nutritionally poor foods. We are also less inclined to move as much and therefore use fewer calories.

Manage stress – the body struggles to metabolise fat as fuel when we are stressed. This makes sense when we consider that raised cortisol levels are part of our fight or flight response. When we're in this state, our body is preparing to fight or run away, both of which require our main focus to be on fuelling the working muscles. So, we divert away from our digestive system, and we call on our rapid sources of energy – carbohydrates. The body will hold onto its fat stores as a protective measure. This is all very well if there's a clear and present danger but, for most of us, stress is chronic in nature and not an immediate response to a real threat.

Keep a food diary – most of us under-estimate how many calories we consume and over-estimate how many calories we expend in a day. Keeping a food diary can help us to get a clear picture of how many calories we're actually eating. Part of the reason we under-estimate is due to mindless eating as mentioned above. There are some good apps available that can help you to track including the My Fitness Pal app or you could simply keep a notebook and pen handy and write down what you're eating manually. You'd be surprised how much you're possibly eating without realising and the very act of writing it down can help to reduce calorie intake.

Nutritional Supplements

If you're eating a good variety of different plant-based foods and a range of protein and healthy fats, nutritional supplements shouldn't really be necessary. However, as we can't always be sure of where our food comes from or how long it has been in transit, there are a few supplements that I would suggest for women during their peri-menopause and beyond.

Multi-vitamin – A good quality, all round multi-vitamin can fill any nutritional gaps – however the key is in the name 'supplement'. A multi-vitamin can't make up for a poor diet.

Omega 3 – fatty acids found in fish oils may help with mild depressive symptoms as well as hot flushes and joint pain. In addition, some studies suggest that fish oils can help with cognitive function and a reduction in the risk of heart disease.

Vitamin B12 – it may be worth taking a vitamin B12 supplement, as B12 is difficult to get in sufficient amounts through diet alone. Many women find they are deficient in B12, especially if they don't eat meat or dairy. B12 can help with insomnia, fatigue, bone health and cognition. You may wish to take a B-Complex vitamin that contains Vitamin B6, B9 and B12 to ensure you are getting the full range of B vitamins.

Vitamin D3 and Calcium – Our modern lifestyles, low sunshine levels in the UK and fear around skin cancer means that we are rarely likely to get sufficient Vitamin D from the sun alone. Vitamin D is essential for helping calcium to get into our bones, and since falling oestrogen levels can increase the risk of osteoporosis, maintaining bone health is essential as we get older. Taking a Vitamin D3 supplement combined with a calcium supplement may help support bone health.

As with herbal supplements, it is best to get an expert opinion before taking vitamin supplements, especially if you have any existing medical conditions. Speak to your GP or to a nutritional therapist to ensure there are no contraindications.

Exercise

I often get asked 'what is the best form of exercise for menopause?' and the simple answer is, whatever exercise you're likely to stick to and do consistently.

However, there are certain activities that I would strongly recommend, particularly for women as they enter peri-menopause and beyond. These include activities that have a positive impact on bone density.

During peri-menopause and particularly post-menopause, reduced oestrogen levels can cause bones to become brittle, a condition known as osteoporosis as we discussed earlier. It is advisable for ALL women (at any age) to include exercise that puts stress on the bones. This is known as 'osteogenic loading' or more commonly 'bone loading' and it is during this process of putting the bone under stress that the cells in the bone renew.

Bone loading can happen with any exercise that places stress on the bones including activities where there is impact (eg jumping, jogging, brisk walking) or resistance (eg weight lifting or bodyweight exercises such as press ups).

Exercises such as swimming and cycling are great for improving cardiovascular health but will have little effect on bone strength, therefore it is advisable for women to include a range of strength and cardiovascular exercise into their weekly regimen.

For women who have never done any formal exercise it can be daunting to begin a new exercise programme. The trick is to begin gently and gradually increase the intensity, duration and type of activity.

The World Health Organisation suggests that we should all be doing a minimum of 150 minutes of moderate exercise or 75 minutes of vigorous exercise per week for good health. In an era where life expectancy is getting longer each year, remaining fit and active in midlife and beyond is becoming more important than ever before.

At a practical level you might think about having walking meetings, getting business done out in nature rather than stuck in a stuffy meeting room. Who says decisions have to be made sitting down! Making use of breaks and lunchtime to get out for a walk or a jog, or incorporating desk exercises such as stretching, press ups and squats can all help. Look up desk yoga on Youtube.

Ideally you want to incorporate activities that cover all

of the components of fitness including:

- Cardiovascular Exercise (also known as aerobic exercise)
- Strength
- Endurance
- Power
- Balance
- Coordination
- Flexibility
- Agility

Different types of exercise will hit different components of fitness. Including a variety of activities will help.

Exercises that help with cardiovascular fitness include walking, jogging, swimming, cycling, dancing, aerobics classes – in fact anything that gets your heart rate up, your breathing rate increased and your body temperature raised.

Exercises that help with strength, endurance, power and agility include things like weight training, circuit training, High Intensity Interval Training (HIIT) and boxing classes.

Flexibility, strength and endurance can be improved with yoga, pilates and other classes that focus on these components including some dance classes.

Dancing and sport can help with coordination and balance.

Everyday activities can also help to increase elements of our fitness including housework, gardening, shopping etc. Think of ways you can incorporate the components of fitness into everyday activities. For example running upstairs, parking farther away from the entrance to the supermarket, grabbing a basket rather than a trolly, taking stairs rather than a lift or escalator, walking or cycling rather than taking the car. You might also want to consider a rise and fall desk so that you can vary your posture between standing and sitting throughout the day.

If you do a desk job, try and factor in some regular breaks. Get up and walk around for 5 minutes, do a few desk stretches and then return to what you're doing.

If you are absolutely brand new to exercise you may want to consider investing in a few sessions with a personal trainer. There are many PTs out there these days who are that bit older and have a much better understanding of the impact of age and menopause on the body. Try and find a trainer who has lots of experience working with older populations. I don't mean working with the elderly necessarily but someone used to working with women over 40.

Many women going through their menopause transition struggle with stress incontinence. This can be helped by regularly performing exercises that help to strengthen the pelvic floor. The pelvic floor is like a girdle of muscles that support the internal organs including the uterus, bladder and intestines. They are involved in the avoidance of urinary and faecal incontinence as well as helping to avoid leakage when put under strain such as when coughing, jumping and heavy lifting.

Pelvic floor exercises can be done anywhere and can be done discretely.

Imagine trying to stop yourself from weeing mid flow. You want to be able to feel the muscles in the pelvic area pulling up towards your belly button. Try to keep all other muscles relaxed – you shouldn't see any external movement if you're doing the pelvic floor exercises correctly. Look out for your bum clenching or your thighs tightening.

You can check if you're accessing the right muscles by inserting 2 fingers into the vagina and squeezing. If you can feel the vagina tightening around your fingers you're probably doing it right. Once you've mastered which muscles to contract, try and do 10 to 15 squeezes every couple of hours. As you get stronger you can aim to hold each squeeze for a few seconds before relaxing and going again.

Sleep and Stress

Night sweats, hot flushes, insomnia, anxiety, panic attacks and poor digestion are all menopause symptoms that can impact on a woman's ability to get a good night's sleep.

Women often complain that fatigue is the hardest symptom of all to deal with. When we are fatigued our stress levels are higher, our concentration is reduced, brain fog increases and self-confidence goes down.

On top of that, when we're tired we tend to reach for sugary, high energy foods which create a rapid increase in blood sugar, followed fairly quickly by a rapid drop which then leaves us feeling even more tired leading to a vicious cycle of highs and lows.

Where stress and anxiety are an issue, women will often self-medicate with alcohol in order to wind down in the evening or to try to induce sleep. Sadly this is counter-productive, since alcohol inhibits the body's ability to reach the deep, restorative levels of sleep needed to help us wake up feeling refreshed.

Oftentimes women will use caffeine as a tool to help with low energy levels during the day. Having tea and coffee or caffeinated carbonated drinks such as cola or even worse, energy drinks, in an attempt to boost energy levels.

Again, this is simply a short-term fix since caffeine can stay in the bloodstream for many hours and, as a stimulant, can inhibit sleep too.

Limiting or eliminating alcohol and caffeine can help with poor sleep, although it is not advisable to cut out caffeine in one go as withdrawal symptoms such as severe headaches can feel worse than the lack of sleep.

Here are some tips to help with poor sleep:

- Aim to keep to a regular sleep routine – going to bed and getting up at the same time each day
- Keep the bedroom cool but draught free
- Invest in natural fabrics for bedding and night clothes
- Avoid using backlit devices such as mobile phones and tablets for an hour before bed as the blue light can affect melatonin production
- Consider supplementing with magnesium as it can help to promote sleep
- Have a warm bath (a hot bath can often trigger flushes) to help relax before bed
- Keep a journal by the bed and write down anything that is playing on your mind before you go to sleep
- Use an app such as Calm or Headspace to help induce a sense of relaxation and to help you clear your mind as you fall asleep.

Stress

I know we often talk about the negative effects of stress, but stress, in reality, is a very good thing. Our stress response, often termed our 'fight or flight' response, is the very thing that has kept us alive and thriving as a species for millennia. And our body is very good at handling acute stress.

When our body is put into a situation where we need to protect ourselves, our adrenal glands release hormones that trigger a range of physical reactions in readiness for us to either fight our way out of trouble or to run away pretty quickly.

Once the danger has passed, our hormones settle back down to baseline levels and normal service is resumed.

At least that is how it should work. Unfortunately, in the modern world in which we live we can't always fight or flee the stressors we encounter. In a world where our stressors are chronic our stress response often remains in a chronically raised state too.

For many women (and men too for that matter) midlife can create a perfect storm of stress, as work, family, financial and health pressures collide.

People reaching middle age right now (however you term middle age) are often referred to as the 'sandwich generation', sandwiched between aging parents often needing extensive care due to medical issues, and children, both young and older, who also need support.

For many women these stresses can be exacerbated by the pressures of a full-time job, often at senior levels, domestic commitments and then, on top of it all, physical and psychological changes that they may or may not recognise as being menopause related.

Imagine a bucket into which we pour life's stresses. In goes our genetic predisposition to how we manage stress. For some this will half fill the bucket before we even get started. Add to that family and domestic stresses. Then pour in financial stress, followed by work stress and maybe relationship stress and that bucket is getting pretty full.

Then, just when you think there's no room left in the bucket, along comes peri-menopause and tips the bucket contents over the edge.

If we don't find a way to put a tap into the bucket to help drain off some of life's stressors our bucket is indeed likely to overflow. And when the bucket overflows, we stop being able to do the things we used to be able to do and our performance in all areas of life goes down.

So what can be done to deal with some of the contents of the bucket?

Where possible, eliminating the stressor is the best solution. Taking time to look at all of the things that we are stressing about, writing them down and taking an honest look at them can help to identify which ones we can remove.

Women, in particular, are very good at taking on too much and feeling responsible for everything and everyone. But when the bucket is full, it is time to start saying no or delegating to others.

Ask, are you expecting too much of yourself?

All too often we take on more than we have capacity for because we don't like saying no. We assume responsibility for things that we aren't responsible for – such as other people's problems.

Here are some tips to help manage stress:
- Write down everything that you have to do and prioritise which are the most important things.
- Once you have your priorities, identify which ones you can eliminate or delegate.
- Ask for help - you don't have to do everything yourself.
- Work out your boundaries – what are you willing and unwilling to accept - and stick to them.

- Practice saying no – decline politely but stick to your boundaries.
- Confide in someone – a problem shared is, indeed, a problem halved.
- Explore new ways of working, maybe utilising technology, to help manage time and aid organisation – often as we enter peri-menopause brain fog means our concentration and memory aren't as good as they used to be. We may need to find strategies to help.
- Take time out for yourself – get some fresh air, go for a walk, have a relaxing bath – whatever feels good for you.
- Take a break from social media or unfollow those who make you feel bad about what's going on in your life.
- Consider CBT if stress is causing anxiety, worry or depression.
- Keep a notebook next to your bed and do a 'brain dump' of everything that's worrying you before you go to sleep.

Have regular one to ones with your manager if you're struggling at work. If you don't feel you can speak to your manager, try to identify someone in work that you can talk to. Maybe you have access to mental health first aiders or to an employee assistance programme where you can ask for help.

Often talking the issues through is enough to dilute them and help you get things in perspective.

Stress is often a feeling of overwhelm and not being in control. Sometimes we have to recognise that things are outside of our control and let go of them.

Imagine you have 3 buckets in front of you. One is labelled 'Full Control' one is labelled 'Some Control' and one is labelled 'No Control'. Now think of all the things you're stressing about, however big or small, and honestly consider which bucket they should go in.

You could even do this for real, writing down each issue on a post–it note and sticking it on one of 3 flipchart sheets each with a different bucket drawn on it!

Things within your control might include losing weight, getting help for menopause symptoms from your GP, saying no to additional tasks, taking a lunch break, delegating some of your tasks.

Things where you have some control might include asking other people for help (you can ask but you can't control if they give it or not), your menopause symptoms (you may be able to reduce them or minimise their impact but you may not be able to eliminate them fully), suggesting alternative working patterns (you may be able to negotiate some changes, but some may not be possible), what you read or see in the media (although you do have full control over what you choose to believe or react to!).

Then there are the things you cannot control, the stuff that needs to go into the 3rd bucket – other people's opinions, other people's actions, the inevitability of getting older and going through menopause, world events, loved ones dying.

Letting go of the things you can't control is incredibly empowering and frees up your brain space to focus only on the things you do have control over. And here is the thing, if you know you have control, then you have no cause to stress.

Thoughts and Feelings

Often women struggling with menopause symptoms such as poor concentration, anxiety, hot flushes and memory issues can begin to question their ability and competence. In the majority of cases these worries are unfounded.

I remember when I was working for the MOD I was certain I was failing in my role and regularly, to my acute embarrassment at the time, found myself in my boss' office in tears convinced he must have thought he'd made a dreadful choice in hiring me!

He always reassured me that it was just my own perception and he had absolutely no concerns about my performance.

It can be exhausting for a woman if she is struggling with brain fog as she will no doubt feel like she's having to work twice as hard to do the things she always took for granted pre- menopause.

This is again where CBT may be helpful as it can help women to understand how their personal thoughts and feelings about menopause and aging in general affect their behaviour.

Other methodologies such as Neurolinguistic Programming (NLP) may also help. A NLP practitioner can help uncover any underlying or unhelpful beliefs that a person may have and provide tools and techniques to help reframe unhelpful thoughts.

Our thoughts and feelings, often known as our mindset, can sometimes feel out of our control. We may believe that our thoughts control us. But the truth is, we can develop control over our thoughts and feelings. In this section I'm going to share a few ideas to help you understand how to become more aware of your thoughts and feelings and how to make them work for you rather than against you.

How we feel about menopause and ageing can have a profound effect on the way we experience our menopause transition.

We often impose many rules about how we should or should not be, or what we should or should not do.

Often we find ourselves saying things like:

I should be doing the ironing

I have to clean the kitchen before I go to bed

I should lose weight

I should know more about menopause and how to deal with it

I have to put my family before myself

We may find ourselves riddled with guilt if we can't be or do the things we think we SHOULD or HAVE to do.

You might have heard the tongue in cheek saying 'stop shoulding all over yourself'!

The truth is that many of the stresses we have in our lives are self-induced and are based around deeply held beliefs that most probably aren't true.

Making a simple shift from SHOULD to COULD helps to take away much of the guilt and stress. Imagine switching the word should for the word could to the statements above.

I could be doing the ironing

I could clean the kitchen

I could lose weight

You get the picture. When you change should to could suddenly it puts you in charge. It becomes a choice rather than an obligation.

Dealing with Negative Self Talk

Have you ever found yourself being really horrible – to yourself?

We often beat ourselves up and talk to ourselves in a way we would NEVER talk to someone else. What may be a perfectly acceptable small scale mistake for others can become a huge catastrophic blunder for us.

You're such an idiot – no wonder you're such a failure.

Who do you think you are anyway, who's going to listen to what you have to say, idiot.

Blimey you look a complete state, why are you such a mess?

Let's face it there's no way you can achieve that, so you might as well give up now.

Many of us have done this all through our lives to some extent, but many women find that their negative self-talk increases as they enter peri-menopause, further adding to their loss of confidence and self-esteem.

The words we use when we talk to ourselves are IMMENSELY powerful. In Neuro Linguistic Programming, practitioners work with their clients to help them identify negative patterns of thought and reframe them to more positive ones.

It is about using language that triggers different emotional responses.

For example you could reframe "Let's face it there's no way you can achieve that, so you might as well give up now."

to

"I probably won't get everything right first time but I'll give it my best shot, and if things don't go as planned, I'll definitely be able to learn from them and be better next time."

Or maybe a more relevant example might be changing

74

"Oh no, I can feel a hot flush coming on, everyone is going to think I'm weird" to "OK, I can feel a hot flush coming on, it's perfectly normal for a woman to have hot flushes and it won't affect my ability to do my job".

Better still, being up front and open about what is happening will help take the pressure off too.

The problem with negative self-talk is that it's insidious.

We often don't realise we're doing it. We run on automatic thought patterns and unless we create a greater self-awareness, catch ourselves doing it and actively reframe the self-talk, it can be hard to stop.

Our thoughts create our emotional response, which then creates our behaviours.

Here's a personal example.

If I think of a snake I create an emotional response of fear and disgust. I feel my hands start to get sweaty and my heart race and that's just thinking about a snake, not even seeing one.

This in turn leads to a certain behaviour.

In my case I feel myself physically shrink as if trying to make myself small so it won't see me. If it was a real snake I'd run away, or more likely, I'd probably pass out!

For others without an issue around snakes, the thought of one creates a different emotional state – it might be one of fascination, whereby their behaviour is about curiosity and they might want to get up close and personal to touch or stroke the snake (OK now I'm really feeling my palms getting sweaty).

Of course, the snake is just a snake. It has no meaning other than the meaning we give it.

For example, I give the snake a meaning of being scary

and dangerous, but others may give it a meaning of strange and fascinating.

So, if our thoughts about ourselves are negative, we get into an emotional state based on those thoughts and behave accordingly.

It's the same with our hot flush scenario above. The hot flush has no meaning other than the meaning we give it.

If our thoughts are negative and we think people are going to be making fun of us, our thoughts will lead to feelings of embarrassment and humiliation. This might cause us to feel anxious which will in turn change our physical response. Our heart might start racing, we might start to feel more sweaty as our stress response kicks in. The result? An even more intense hot flush.

These thought patterns create a kind of self-fulfilling prophecy because chances are now, instead of the hot flush being barely noticeable, we've exaggerated the body's response and drawn even more attention to it.

Therefore, if we can change the meaning, we can change our response.

The good news is that we do have control of our thoughts and therefore our feelings, IF we are aware of them.

We tend to think in words, pictures, sounds, smells, taste – basically our internal language is a mixture of different representational systems. Certain smells or sounds can elicit a particular emotional response too.

For example, when I pass a coffee shop with a strong aroma of freshly brewed coffee I'm immediately transported in my head to my teenage years, walking through Fenwick's Department Store in Newcastle. It brings back happy memories of enjoyable shopping trips with my friends and creates a happy emotional state. This is known as anchoring and I've anchored a happy feeling to the smell of freshly brewed coffee.

You can simulate an anchor in order to anchor feelings of confidence for example, to call upon when you feel an anxious thought creeping in.

Here's what you need to do.

Close your eyes and imagine a time when you felt supremely confident (or whatever feeling you want recreate). Fully immerse yourself in those feelings.

What can you see, smell, hear, taste, and feel. Make the feeling as strong as possible. Imagine the feelings in bright, vibrant colours. Put yourself fully into the centre of the memory.

Rather than imagining yourself looking at yourself being confident, imagine jumping inside of your body and really BEING the you that felt supremely confident. This is called being in an 'associated' state.

When you feel you're fully immersed in that supremely confident feeling, squeeze your little finger tightly for a few seconds. As the strength of the memory begins to fade, release your grip on your little finger.

Give everything a bit of a shake for a minute and maybe focus on something completely different (this is known as 'breaking state') before closing your eyes and conjuring up that feeling of confidence once again. Make it as bright and vibrant as you can, be fully associated in the memory and when you feel yourself reaching the peak of that feeling, squeeze your little finger again.

Repeat the process a few more times.

You can test the anchor by squeezing your little finger

and noticing if you get that feeling of confidence come back. If you don't feel it too strongly, repeat the anchoring process a few more times and test again.

Then, whenever you want to feel confident in the future, maybe when you feel a hot flush coming on, you can grab that little finger and give it a squeeze.

You'll have anchored a feeling of confidence into your unconscious mind and be able to get into that confident state immediately.

The more you use the anchor, the stronger it will get.

Taking Responsibility for Our Outcomes

Learning to become more self-aware and challenging our negative thoughts gives us the opportunity to reframe the thoughts and this leads to a different response and ultimately a different outcome.

Use this simple equation: $E + R = O$

Quite simply this means an Event (something outside of our control) plus our Response (which is within our control) = The Outcome.

Here's a quick example.

Imagine you're driving in the middle lane of the motorway and a young man in a black BMW comes flying down the outside lane and cuts in sharply in front of you.

That's an Event over which you have no control.

Now imagine your thoughts about that event go something like: "what a total idiot. Who does he think he is. Typical BMW driver they think they rule the road. I'll show him…"

Those thoughts may trigger emotions of anger and indignation and therefore your Reponse might be to speed up and get right behind him to PROVE that he's not intimidating you, you might flash your lights angrily or beep your horn to 'teach him a lesson'.

Then, imagine you realise that in your distracted state you're going to miss your exit slip road so you quickly move over just to find that you failed to see the car in your blind spot on your driver side – CRUNCH!

Mr BMW driver is now continuing on his merry way totally oblivious to the fact he's annoyed you and now you're responsible for an accident.

Event + Response = Outcome

So how about if you reframed the event.

What if you took control of your thoughts and they went more like "ooh that was a bit close, his driving is a bit reckless, but no harm done."

These thoughts trigger a less volatile emotional Response.

You're not distracted by trying to 'teach him a lesson', you're more focused and relaxed and when you see your exit slip road you have more time to check behind you to make sure it's safe to move over.

The outcome – NO ACCIDENT. Not to mention less stress.

Event + Response = Outcome

Looking at those two different scenarios. Who do you think is Responsible for the accident?

The driver of the car you crashed into certainly won't be blaming the BMW driver!

So you see, even though we often think we don't have control of how we think and feel, we always have a choice, we just have to be more self-aware.

Listen out for your own negative self-talk and become more aware of how your thoughts may be creating negative outcomes for you.

Coaching is a great way to help you to see where your own beliefs and thoughts may be holding you back.

One of my favourite sayings is 'You can't read the label from inside of the jar'.

A coach can help you to look at your own beliefs, values and attitudes from a different perspective, which is incredibly empowering.

This is especially true when it comes to our beliefs about menopause, the role of women in society and particularly the way we think about getting older.

If you'd like to discuss how coaching could help you build confidence, manage your menopause more effectively or simply help you to feel less anxious and perform better, you can email me bev@florescotraining.co.uk for an initial conversation, to find out if coaching is right for you and to see if we would be a good fit to work together.

Dealing with Loss

For some women menopause can feel like a major relief. No more periods, no more risk of unwanted pregnancy, no more having to remember to take birth control measures and no more having to worry too much about what other people think.

Conversely, many women struggle with menopause because it feels like an uncontrollable loss. This can often feel like a grieving process. Alongside the physical and hormonal changes that occur during the menopause transition, for many women, especially those in the normal menopausal age bracket of 45 to 55, there are myriad other changes that may be occurring.

These could include 'empty nest syndrome' as children cut the apron strings and set out on their own, leaving the family home feeling quiet and bare. This can often lead to a sense of lost identity as the role of nurturing mother and homemaker is needed less. This can create conflicting emotions – on the one hand a recognition of a job well done and potentially more time to oneself, on the other hand a sense of mourning for something that you can never get back.

In addition, often during this time women are caring for elderly parents and may be dealing with the loss of loved ones.

Women often say they lose their libido and lose any sense of their sexuality. Intimacy is challenging as body changes, poor sleep, lethargy and low self-esteem take hold. They may feel a sense of loss of youth. A sense that they are no longer attractive or desirable. Women often say they don't get the same strength of orgasm and are sometimes left feeling frustrated, angry or sad.

For women who have struggled to conceive, the onset of menopause can be devastating as they feel their time has run out. Even women who don't actually want to have more children can feel saddened at the prospect that their choice has been taken from them.

For women who experience an early menopause in their 20s or 30s this loss can be even more significant and may feel totally devastating.

On top of all this, society doesn't do a great job of 'bigging up' older women. The pervading perception that older women are 'over the hill' or 'past their best' is a narrative that needs to be challenged. The best way for that to happen is for women themselves to stand tall and stand up for who and what they are and not allow themselves to become invisible.

The Change Curve

In her book 'Death and Dying', psychiatrist Elisabeth Kubler-Ross introduced a model for understanding the emotional process we experience as we come to terms with loss known as 'The Change Curve'. Also sometimes referred to as 'The 5 Stages of Grief', this model has since been adopted by many coaches, counsellors and leaders as a way to help people deal with change.

Let's look in detail at each of the 5 stages of the Change Curve:

1. **Denial:** This is the first stage and is usually accompanied by shock and disbelief. We can feel angry and dismiss any evidence that we don't want to believe. There is no set timescale involved here, some people may move through denial quickly and onto the next phase while others struggle to move on, taking more of a 'head in the sand' approach.

2. **Anger:** Once a person has acknowledged that a change is indeed taking place they may become angry and look for someone to blame. In the case of menopause this can, in itself, cause emotional turmoil since there is no one to blame. This feeling of anger may be expressed as frustration, irritability or quick temper and is often based on an underlying feeling of fear.

3. **Bargaining:** In this stage, having realised there is no one to blame, we may turn our attention to ourselves or to something greater than ourselves. 'Please, God, don't let this be happening to me'. Part

of the bargaining phase may be to try to fight against the change, throwing ourselves into any number of radical health regimes, pills and potions to try to fend off the inevitable and buy us time.

4. Depression: When we feel that our bargaining is getting us nowhere and that we actually can't prevent the change from occurring, we may enter a period of depression. We may feel a sense of hopelessness or overwhelm. We may wonder 'what's the point' and find ourselves withdrawing from our social groups, becoming lethargic and lacking motivation for life.

5. Acceptance: The final stage of the change curve is acceptance. This is where we start to feel ready to move forward, to make plans and feel more optimistic. We may not be happy about the change, but we've accepted the inevitability of it and stopped fighting it. We may start to feel the depression begin to lift and feel more ready to face the world again. We may start to feel our self-confidence rising, the lethargy lessening and our sense of self returning.

Everyone is unique and will move through the stages of the change curve at different rates. For some they may even miss a stage, for others it may feel like they're constantly moving backwards and forwards between stages – and this is all very normal.

Ultimately we want to get to the Acceptance stage as quickly as we can in a timescale that feels right for us. Talking with a coach or a therapist can certainly help as can sharing experiences in a group with others going through menopause too.

Often just realising that what we are feeling is normal and knowing that it is a stage in a process, can be a big help.

Whatever stage you're currently at I want you to remember one important fact:

YOU ARE PERFECTLY NORMAL!

CHAPTER 7

> To be passive is to let others decide for you. To be aggressive is to decide for others. To be assertive is to decide for yourself. And to trust that there is enough, that you are enough.

Edith Eva Eger

7 Preparing for a visit to your GP

For the majority of women heading towards menopause, a trip to the GP is very likely.

When you choose to make that appointment will depend on a number of factors including the severity of your symptoms, your level of knowledge (which hopefully having come this far through this book will now be high) and other personal circumstances.

What often happens is that we book our 10-minute appointment with the GP, we go in to the appointment unprepared and come away feeling disappointed with the outcome.

We ask a great deal of our GPs – as general practitioners they are expected to know an awful lot about an awful lot and at the end of the day they are only human. Unfortunately, unless a GP has chosen to undertake specialist training into modern menopause treatment options he or she is likely to have limited up-to-date knowledge.

You can improve your chances of getting a solution that is right for you by doing your own research before you even make your appointment.

A good place to start is by keeping a journal of your symptoms. You can download a simple symptom checklist from the resources section at the end of this book, which will help you to determine whether the symptoms you are experiencing are likely to be menopause related or not.

Bear in mind that symptoms of menopause may also be symptoms of other conditions, but by keeping track of your particular symptoms your GP will be able to look at what you're experiencing as a whole and therefore make a more accurate diagnosis.

Often what happens is women visit their GP unprepared, focus on just one symptom and the GP is then making a diagnosis on limited information.   Therefore, the more comprehensive a picture you give, the more likely you are to get the right outcome.

I would suggest keeping a symptom journal for one month. Note down any symptoms, the time of day and any external events that may have been happening just before you noticed the symptom.

Next assess how severe each symptom is. Using a simple scale between 1 to 10, where 1 is barely noticeable at all and 10 is absolutely horrendous and leaves you feeling wiped out, make a subjective judgement about the symptom's severity.

Then think about the impact your symptoms are having on your life. Consider the impact on your relationships, your self-esteem and confidence, you family, your performance in work, your social life and your sex life.

When you've collated a month's worth of data, look back and see if you can identify the 3 or 4 main symptoms that are causing you problems.   Create a one-page document (either typed or hand-written) that you can take with you to your GP so that you have something to remind you of what you want to discuss.

Invariably we can end up becoming emotional as we try to talk to the GP and forget to mention some key points. By having your notes with you, you will feel much more in control and more likely to get a positive outcome.

Before your appointment do some research into the treatment options you feel would be right for you.   And be prepared to ask specifically for what you want.   There are some very good resources available to help you make an informed decision about the type of hormone replacement therapy you might prefer. Consider visiting the patient arm of the British Menopause Society's website called the 'Women's Health Concern' for accurate, up to date information on HRT. You could also visit the NHS website. You can also rely on the information in Chapter 5 to help you make your decision about your preferences for managing your menopause.

Your GP is far more likely to agree to prescribing your chosen option if he or she can see that you've already done your research and you are clear on the risks and benefits associated with your choice. However, you may come across a GP who simply isn't willing to prescribe what you are asking for.

If there are medical reasons why HRT is not a good option for you then your GP should explain that to you. Although there are, in fact, very few situations where HRT is an absolute no and if you feel that you're not being given good advice, you may wish to seek out the opinion of an alternative GP or speak to a specialist menopause practitioner.

It may therefore be prudent to ask when making your appointment, who within the practice has done further specialist menopause training, or at least ask who within the practice has an interest in menopause. Don't make the assumption that a female doctor will necessarily know more or be more sympathetic than a male doctor.

Many women feel they would like to be given a blood test to confirm whether or not they have started peri–menopausal or have reached menopause. For women who have been taking contraception that stopped their periods they may find it difficult to know if they're in menopause or not.

Please note that the current NICE guidelines in England do not advise the use of blood tests to diagnose menopause for women over 45. GPs are advised to make their diagnosis based on symptoms and an assessment of any other medical conditions. A single blood test is unlikely to give a true picture since during peri-menopause hormone levels can fluctuate significantly and therefore a single blood test will only give a snap-shot of hormone levels on that particular day.

For women under 45, a series of blood tests may be advised in order to rule peri-menopause in or out.

Elaine's Story

At the age of 46, I suddenly started getting migraines and horrific mood swings every month. I had suffered from migraines periodically over the years and they were always stress induced but this felt like something new. I had not suffered with mood swings since being a teenager but this wasn't the kind of "turning back the clock" experience I wanted!

It took a couple of months to realise they were happening every month at about the same time and they were getting steadily more debilitating.

I changed back to my usual contraceptive pill (having been prescribed a different one by a new doctor as mine was out of stock) and this seemed to reduce the regularity and ferocity for a while but it didn't last. In the meantime I had started taking evening primrose oil to combat the mood swings – wonderful stuff for me and I still take it daily for everybody's' sanity!

About eight months ago, I started to notice a couple of other symptoms; the occasional hot flush and brain fog – oh the struggle to actually form the words I had in my head!

So, recently I decided to book an appointment with a GP to discuss options.

I didn't want to come off the pill (until I have to) but the migraines have got to the stage where I lose 3 to 4 days a month unable to do anything at all and I am getting pretty hacked off with my lack of word recall. I have to admit that I did ask for a female GP and she was very pragmatic. She listened to my issues (although in true brain fog fashion I forgot to mention the brain fog, leaving the list I had prepared in my handbag...!) and discussed various options. We agreed that HRT probably wasn't necessary at this stage as my combined pill is probably masking some of the symptoms.

I am now in receipt of a prescription of progestogen only pill (POP) which I start taking on Friday with the directive that "we are just waiting for trouble to start after that"! On the plus side, she did seem to think that it may help regulate the hormonal changes each month, hopefully having a positive impact on my migraine habit.

My take aways so far, having spoken to many women who are at this stage of life, my mum and read lots of helpful literature are: Eat well, move lots, sleep lots, do more of what makes you happy, be aware of your body and don't be afraid to ask for help.

I have no idea what path my journey will take going forward, only time will tell – watch this space!

CHAPTER 8

> " Our mothers were largely silent about what happened to them as they passed through this midlife change. But a new generation of women has already started to break the wall of silence. "

Trisha Posner

8 Menopause and the Workplace

Go back not that many years and no one would have been talking about menopause as a workplace issue. It was, and in some organisations still is, a taboo subject. A subject that could make men squirm and women rush off to find the nearest hole to jump into.

Thankfully times are changing and more and more organisations are recognising the need to offer support and understanding to their female workforce. And this isn't just a nice thing to do (although of course it is the RIGHT thing to do!).

The role of women in the workplace is changing rapidly, with women over the age of 50 currently the fastest growing sector of the UK workforce.

If we look back just 25 years, the number of women aged 50 plus in work has increased 72% and there are currently 4.4 million women in this age group in work (as at 2019).

It is also reported that 75-80% of women going through their menopause transition are working but that a shocking 25% of women have considered leaving their job due to a lack of support or feeling unable to ask for help for fear of judgement.

What Are My Rights as a Woman Going Through Menopause?

In terms of the Equality Act 2010 menopause is not, in itself, a protected characteristic. However, since the menopause is primarily an issue that affects women, there is certainly a gender issue here.

It needs to be remembered that symptoms related to menopause and hormone imbalance can affect non-binary people and trans men as well as women.

Under The Equality Act 2010 (in the UK) employers must not discriminate on the grounds of either age or gender and must ensure that all employees are treated with respect and not unfairly disadvantaged .

In addition, whilst menopause is not in itself a disability, where symptoms have a long term and substantial adverse effect on a person's ability to perform their day-to-day activities, this condition may be deemed a disability under the Equality Act and reasonable adjustments should be considered to help the individual get their performance back up to an acceptable level. Failure to do so could (and has) leave an organisation liable to a claim on the grounds of discrimination.

It is clear that whilst menopause may not be a protected characteristic, the nature of menopause means that it is likely to be covered under anti-discrimination laws relating to age, sex and disability.

If you feel you have been discriminated against or unfairly treated as a direct result of your menopause you may wish to seek advice from your trades union representative, your line manager or your human resources department.

Ideally your employer will have clear menopause guidance or a specific menopause policy which lays out the responsibilities of employers, managers and colleagues in relation to menopause. In reality, however, only a small number of employers at the time of writing this book actually have a formalised policy or guidance.

Regardless of whether guidance is in place, your employer does have a duty of care to ensure your health and safety and as such is required to treat you fairly, without discrimination and in a way that supports you to perform to the best of your ability.

This may include enabling reasonable adjustments to be made to your working conditions and also carrying out risk assessments to ensure that you and those you work with are working as safely as possible.

If you need support, your first port of call would ideally be with your direct line manager. Here are some things to consider before speaking to your boss:

- What are your main symptoms?
- What impact are they having on you – both at home and at work?
- What steps have you taken already to address your issues (eg seen a GP, addressed lifestyle factors etc)?
- What are the main difficulties specifically related to your workplace?
- What changes (reasonable adjustments) would help?
- Specifically, what help are you asking for?

A good employer (and a good boss) will listen with empathy and without judgment and be prepared to meet reasonable requests for support. In the majority of cases, adjustments are short term and low cost. You may need to be prepared to compromise since your manager will have to balance what is reasonable to meet your needs with what is reasonable to meet the business' needs.

If you don't feel you have a good enough relationship with your manager to be able to talk to him or her about menopause, consider if there is someone else within the organisation that you can approach to seek help. This may be your HR department, a trusted colleague, a women's health champion, occupational health or a mental health first aider.

Remember, menopause is a natural part of a woman's

life cycle that EVERY WOMAN will go through if she lives beyond 60 years or so. There is no need to feel embarrassed or stigmatised by menopause.

There are very many adjustments that may be made to support you to remain happy and productive throughout your menopause transition. It is not possible to cover every scenario, particularly as each individual will experience menopause in a unique way and will have a unique situation. However, in the table below I've laid out some common reasonable adjustments and the symptoms they relate to:

Hot Flushes	Assess lighting and room temperature. Review seating arrangements and proximity to fresh air. Make desk fans easily available. Consider impact uniform or dress code.
Sleep Disruption	Consider flexible working patterns. Later start/finish times. Work from home options.
Tiredness or Fatigue	Quiet space. Regular breaks. Flexible working patterns.
Fluctuating or Heavy Periods	Access to sanitary products. Easy access to toilet and changing facilities.
Anxiety, Confidence, Panic Attacks	Regular one-to-one discussions. Referral to Occupational Health or Counselling Services.

You may also wish to ask your manager to refer you to Occupational Health who will be able to advise on the best way to manage your menopause within the workplace. In addition, if you have an Employee Assistance Programme, there may be the opportunity to access counselling for Cognitive Behavioural Therapy which has strong evidence to show it can be a very effective tool for managing many of the physical, psychological and emotional symptoms related to menopause.

You may also be able to access funding for coaching to help you overcome some of the difficulties you may be facing in the workplace. These might include low confidence, time management, stress management, loss of identity and self-doubt. Executive coaching with someone who understands menopause and the difficulties that it can bring can be a highly effective, solution focused tool to help you feel more in control. Coaching is not about telling. It is not counselling or training. Coaching is a respectful relationship in which the coach and coachee work together to find solutions to the coachee's problems through exploration, powerful questioning, overcoming self-limiting beliefs and goal setting. To learn more about how we support our clients through coaching email me at bev@florescotraining.co.uk.

Michelle's Story

I'm sure I was peri-menopausal a lot earlier than I realised, and I so wish there was better information available out there, it is improving but there is still too much that is confusing and misleading.

Since about age 45 I began suffering from increasing anxiety, recurring depression, stress, brain fog and overwhelm, lower libido and low mood. I think the brain fog and overwhelm was the worst as I just couldn't multi-task anymore and being able to run my day to day home admin as well as help out with my husband's business was a constant challenge.

I eventually realised when I was turning 50 that this wasn't just another period of depression and stress, it was actually menopause and I needed to try and find help. I wasted a lot of money avoiding going on HRT – having read all the negative press – and not wanting to be judged by others for deciding to take HRT.

I tried exercise and nutrition, I tried a private GP and bio-identical hormones from a compounding pharmacy. Eventually I sought proper help from my specialist menopause GP but it was a slow journey. I was very sensitive to the progesterone, but she was unable to prescribe outside of the NICE guidelines. So, after doing my own research I went to see a private specialist in London and finally got the right combination of HRT in the right doses for me. I am on body identical HRT which can be prescribed on the NHS now thus reducing the cost of private prescriptions.

I would say to any other 45+ women – don't hesitate – trust your instinct and get help earlier. Do your research but HRT is not the horror we have been led to believe and it can be life-changing. It was for me!

Useful Contacts and Resources

Contacts

Floresco Menopause Training and Coaching
www.florescotraining.co.uk

British Menopause Society's Women's Health Concern
www.womens-health-concern.org

Dr Louise Newson
www.menopausedoctor.co.uk

The NHS Website
www.nhs.uk/conditions/menopause

NICE Menopause Guidance
www.nice.org.uk/guidance/NG23

The Daisy Network – Charity for Women with POI
www.daisynetwork.org

The Pleasure Possibility – Dr Claire Macaulay
www.pleasurepossibility.com

The National Institute of Medical Herbalists
www.nimh.org.uk

The Research Council for Complementary Medicine
www.rccm.org.uk

Resources

To download these additional free resources visit my **Freebie Vault** at:

https://bit.ly/bevsfreestuff

Where you'll find a lots of helpful guides, trackers and video trainings in addition to those mentioned in the book.

The Generation Exceptional Podcast – Listen on any of your favourite podcast apps including Apple, Spotify, Google, Amazon and Podbean

Your Best Midlife – Join me in my Facebook world where I share more help and support to women navigating their midlife transition.

Visit https://www.facebook.com/groups/yourbestmidlife

About Me...

I never thought I'd be calling myself an entrepreneur in my mid 50s, but I guess that's what I've somehow found myself becoming.

For over 30 years, I worked a normal job for the British military, first the Army – starting out in the Outer Hebrides off the West Coast of Scotland – then the Royal Air Force, which brought me to the Midlands and into the path of my ever patient husband Mark.

We have 2 grown up kids, 1 sassy little granddaughter and a long succession of fur babies. When I'm not spouting off about menopause, I love nothing more than sticking some jigs and reels on Spotify and bashing along on my Bodhran (pronounced bow-ron it's an Irish frame drum made of wood and goat skin).

Before the big 'M' hit, I had a great life working for the Royal Air Force. We lived in Cyprus for 3 years and brought in the millennium there. The Ministry of Defence put me through my business degree, took me on trips all over Europe studying military history, and brought me the most amazing group of long-term friends and more work pals than I can even begin to recall.

But when I turned 50 in 2016 something shifted in me. For a start, along with the gorgeous birthday cake and huge '50 Today' badge, I also got my first hot flush!

What followed was 2 years of confusion as anxiety, low confidence, brain fog and self-doubt plagued what I had always thought was a pretty steady, normal brain.

Despite my best efforts at getting myself fit and healthy, I struggled to shake off the feeling that I was constantly failing and never close to being enough.

We had a lot going on around that time. Mark was leaving the Air Force after 38 years, my daughter had a traumatic labour and had been in and out of hospital for nearly 2 years and remained undiagnosed and my physically and mentally disabled sister had moved into the house next door to us so that Mark could help to take care of her.

It was the perfect storm, with everything hitting me at once.

Little did I realise that many of my symptoms were menopause related.

After struggling for 2 years I decided to ask for 12 months unpaid leave to help get myself sorted out but sadly, due to financial constraints, my request was rejected.

Feeling somewhat stuck for options, I resigned my job in March 2018.

I set up Floresco Training and Coaching in 2018 to help raise awareness of the impact of menopause on working women. I don't want women to feel as I did, that they have no option than to give up their career because of a lack of education, understanding or support.

Unlike so many women, I actually had an amazing boss, but at the time the MOD offered no awareness training either for colleagues or managers. Consequently, I wasn't aware that many of my issues were menopause related, which meant I didn't ask for the help I probably needed. And even though my boss was great, he had had no training either to help him spot the signals.

Since starting Floresco I've been lucky enough to speak to hundreds of businesses, across all sectors, and thousands of women and colleagues to raise the level of education around this natural period in every woman's life.

I feel passionately that the narrative around menopause and older women has to change. The taboo, stigma and 'hush hush' mentality that pervades around menopause, and indeed women's reproductive health in general, has to go.

I am committed to keeping the menopause conversation going and supporting women to feel positive about this amazing metamorphosis through which every woman, God willing, will pass.

It has been a roller coaster ride over the last few years, and there are simply too many people who have supported me on my journey to mention in this book. However, there are a few for whom I owe a debt of gratitude as I could not have made it this far without them and for that I believe they deserve a special mention.

To my husband and best friend Mark, fixer of all things, applier of sound logic and first-class tea maker, you truly are my rock. To my daughter Amy, thank you for humouring me as I talked endlessly to you about menopause, I just hope I haven't scared you too much. To my son Ben, thank you for your sense of humour and patience every time I've needed 'technical support'!

There are a few more people to whom I am enormously grateful, and the first has to be my friend and ex-work colleague Alison Thompson, if not for you none of the work I'm now doing would have ever happened. To Dr Claire MacCauley for writing the foreword and for pushing me way out of my comfort zone talking 'orgasmic yoga' on the Podcast. To my best friend Diane, for starting this journey with me and gifting me the name of my business 'Floresco', which means simply to flourish and could not be more apt.

To my good friend and font of all knowledge Katy, for always believing in everything I do. To my ever patient business coach David, for listening to all my hair brained ideas and still being able to keep me on track. And finally to Anna Richards for bringing the whole book together and making it happen on time.

Printed in Great Britain
by Amazon